Fluid and Blood Component Therapy in the Critically Ill and Injured

CONTEMPORARY ISSUES IN CRITICAL CARE NURSING — VOL. 1

Forthcoming Volumes in the Series

Fluid and Blood Component Therapy in the Critically Ill and Injured

Edited by

Suellyn Ellerbe, R.N., M.N.

Clinical Assistant Professor
Department of Physiological Nursing
University of Washington
Nursing Director, Burn Center
Harborview Medical Center
Seattle, Washington

Churchill Livingstone
NEW YORK, EDINBURGH, LONDON, AND MELBOURNE 1981

Distributed in the United Kingdom by Churchill Livingstone, Robert Stevenson House, 1-3 Baxter's Place, Leith Walk, Edinburgh EH1 3AF and by associated companies, branches and representatives throughout the world.

First published 1981

Printed in USA

ISBN 0-443-08129-8

7   6   5   4   3   2

Library of Congress Cataloging in Publication Data

Main entry under title:

Fluid and blood component therapy in the
  critically ill and injured.

  (Contemporary issues in critical care
nursing; 1)
  Bibliography: p.
  Includes index.
  1. Fluid therapy. 2. Blood—Transfusion.
3. Intensive care nursing. 4. Critical care
medicine. I. Ellerbe, Suellyn. II. Series.
[DNLM: 1. Fluid therapy—Nursing texts.
2. Blood transfusion—Nursing texts.
3. Critical care—Nursing texts. 4. Wounds
and injuries—Therapy—Nursing texts.
W1 CO769MQM v. 1 no. 1/WY 154 F6461
RM170.F58   615'.39   81-10033
ISBN 0-443-08129-8   AACR2

Contributors

Maribel J. Clements, R.N., M.A.
Clinical Associate, Puget Sound Blood Center, Seattle, Washington

Diane M. Cooper, R.N., B.A., M.N.
Clinical Nurse Specialist, Major Abdominal Surgery, University of California at San Francisco, San Francisco, California

John T. Corpening, R.N., M.N., C.C.R.N., R.R.T
Clinical Nursing Supervisor, Critical Care, Harborview Medical Center, Seattle, Washington

Suellyn Ellerbe, R.N., M.N.
Clinical Assistant Professor, Department of Physiological Nursing, University of Washington, Seattle; Nursing Director, Burn Center, Harborview Medical Center, Seattle, Washington

Mary Farley, R.N., C.C.R.N. (Masters Candidate)
Burn Trauma Emergency Nursing, Department of Physiological Nursing, University of Washington, Seattle, Washington

Margaret M. McMahon, R.N., M.N., CEN, C.C.R.N
Lecturer, Family Nurse Practitioner Program, University of Washington, Seattle; Emergency Medical Services Consultant, Seattle, Washington

Diana L. Nikas, R.N., M.N., C.C.R.N., C.N.R.N.
Assistant Professor, Critical Care Clinical Specialist Program, California State University, Long Beach; Clinical Nurse Specialist, Neurology–Neurosurgery, Los Angeles County–University of Southern California Medical Center, Los Angeles, California

Wanda L. Roberts, R.N., M.N.
Assistant Professor, Department of Physiological Nursing, University of Washington, Seattle; Educational Coordinator, Burn Center, Harborview Medical Center, Seattle, Washington

Foreword

In the time since the first intensive care unit was built over two decades ago, the role of the critical care nurse has evolved to embrace the holistic model of practice. Critical care nurses absorbed in stride the knowledge base and accompanying technical skills that previously had been the jealously guarded territory of the physician. They literally became the lifeline for the critically ill and injured. Soon, however, critical care nurses were forced to cope with the health care ethics that macrotechnology wrought—such as whether to prolong life when the quality of life is questionable, "no code," organ donation, and medical versus legal death, among others. Critical care nurses met these challenges with remarkable resiliency during this initial period of rapidly escalating technology and resultant medicoethical dilemmas.

And what of the future? Volatile medical/social issues such as the right to health care, and the related costs, will predominate in the media and generate heated debate. Regardless of these highly publicized and provocative topics, the now highly evolved critical care nursing specialty will continue to undergo refinement as nurses and hospitals develop standards of care and quality-assurance activities. New technology will require critical care nurses to incorporate new skills into their nursing care practice, and it is safe to assume that new knowledge will be the catalyst for this technology. As the title implies, the purpose of *Contemporary Issues In Critical Care Nursing* is to provide the critical care nurse practitioner with timely and relevant knowledge. The time is right for a publication directed and edited *by* critical care nurses *for* critical care nurses. Carefully chosen (and even controversial) topics will enhance the core knowledge base of the reader in a sophisticated yet easily readable style. *Contemporary Issues In Critical Care Nursing* will serve as a vital resource for enabling the critical care nurse to continue to be the lifeline of the critically ill or injured patient. Your response to this new publication is sincerely encouraged.

John T. Corpening

Contents

Fluid and Blood Component Therapy in the Critically Ill and Injured

1 | Principles of Fluid and Electrolyte Balance and Imbalance

Wanda L. Roberts

At some point in the course of many disease states, disturbances occur in fluid and electrolyte balance. These disturbances can result from cell or tissue changes that are primarily the result of the disease process, from illness-associated changes in the intake of food or fluids, or as a consequence of therapy for the disease. Because of the acute and often extensive physiologic derangements that occur in the critically ill, this group of patients is particularly vulnerable to severe and complex body fluid and electrolyte imbalance. The situation is complicated further by the fact that in the critically ill, the kidneys, the organs principally responsible for regulating the volume and composition of body fluids, often fail to some degree. This makes greater precision in the calculation of fluid and electrolyte losses and the administration of supplements necessary, since the kidneys themselves cannot make the final adjustments for over- or under-compensation of deficits. Failure to recognize or promptly correct fluid and electrolyte disorders in the critically ill can often lead to fatal complications.

Nurses caring for patients with potential or real fluid and electrolyte disturbances must assume a primary monitoring role. This role entails identifying those patients at risk for specific fluid and electrolyte imbalances, as well as the painstaking, continuous observation and analysis of the physiologic indices of fluid and electrolyte balance, so that derangements in these two vital factors can be recognized early, and corrective measures can be instituted. The source and amount of any body-fluid loss, as well as the volume and composition of all exogenously administered fluids, should be recorded judiciously.

Requisite to the proficient implementation of these measures is an understanding of the fundamental concepts of normal fluid and electrolyte composition, distribution, and regulation within the body; of the pathophysiology of body-fluid disturbances; and of the rationale that underlies the medical correction of any imbalance in fluids or electrolytes. These concepts will be outlined in this chapter.

BODY WATER

Volume and Distribution

The total volume of water in the body is expressed as a percentage of body weight, and in adults ranges from 50 to 70 percent of the latter. This variation in range is due mainly to the inverse relationship between body water and fat: since fat contains virtually no water, an obese individual will have a smaller water-percentage of body weight than will a lean person.[1] In young males, the average total water volume is 60 percent of the body weight; in young females, who have a larger amount of body fat than do males, it is 50 percent. With age, the water content of the tissues decreases steadily with the effect that in elderly males and females, the average total water volume constitutes only 52 and 46 percent, respectively,[2] of the body weight. Clinically, calculation of individual fluid and electrolyte needs is based on these average figures for body-water volume.

Water in the body is distributed among two major compartments: the intracellular fluid (ICF) and the extracellular fluid (ECF). The ICF comprises approximately two-thirds of the total body water, with the greatest amount residing in the skeletal muscle. The ECF contains the remaining water, of which one-third is distributed to the plasma or intravascular fluid (IVF) compartment, and the remainder to the interstitial fluid (ISF) compartment. Functionally, the ISF and IVF are in close relationship, and most of the ISF equilibrates rapidly with the plasma. However, the ISF also contains such components as connective tissue water and the so-called transcellular fluids (for example, endocrine-gland, joint, and cerebrospinal fluids) that are much more slow to exchange with the plasma. These latter components account for approximately 10 percent of the total ISF volume.[1,2]

Movement and Composition

Although water distribution in the body is described as having specific compartmental boundaries, it is important to understand that the membranes separating these compartments are freely permeable to water, and that the latter is therefore constantly moving from one compartment to another. The direction and rate of water movement depend mainly upon the total number of particles or solutes (such as electrolytes, nonelectrolytes, and proteins) in each compartment that are capable of attracting water. The amount of "pull" or force created by the random movement of these particles in their respective compartments is termed osmotic pressure. The degree of pressure exerted is proportional to the total number of osmotically active particles dispersed in the body water—the parameter known as osmolality.

The term osmosis refers to the process of water movement across the membrane in response to osmotic pressure. Water always moves from the compartment with the lowest osmotic pressure (the lowest concentration of solutes) toward the compartment with the highest osmotic pressure (the greatest solute concentration); it will do this until the concentration of solutes, relative to the amount of water present, is equal in both compartments. The osmolality of each fluid compartment of the body ranges from 280 to 295 milliosmoles (mOsm) per liter.[3-5] The ionic composition of the body fluids is shown in Figure 1-1. Note that although the ionic composition of each compartment is different, the osmolality of each is the same.

Intracellularly, potassium (K^+) and magnesium (Mg^{2+}) are the principal cations, and phosphates and proteins are the principle anions. In the ECF, sodium (Na^+) is the major osmotically active cation, and chloride (Cl^-) and bicarbonate (HCO_3^-) are the major anions. Because of the abundance of Na^+ in the ECF, movement of fluid between the ECF and ICF—and thus the volume of the ECF compartment—depends chiefly upon the concentration of this ion.

Ionic concentrations are expressed as milliequivalents (mEq) per liter: a parameter that indicates the chemical combining activity of each type of ion. Within each compartment, the sum of the cation milliequivalents equals the sum of the anion milliequivalents—a balance that must be maintained in order for the solution to remain electrically neutral. Normally, the cell membrane, which is relatively impermeable to solutes, maintains the differences in ionic composition that exist for the ICF and ECF.[2] A slightly greater amount of protein exists in the plasma than in the ISF, owing to the relative impermeability of capillaries to protein. This difference is partially offset by a slightly greater concentration of inorganic ions in the ISF than in the plasma.

Movement of isotonic fluid between the IVF and the ISF compartments is influenced by a balance between the capillary hydrostatic pressure—which favors fluid movement from the plasma to the ISF—and the osmotic force exerted by the plasma proteins (the colloid osmotic pressure), which favors movement of fluid in the opposite direction.[6] In a normal steady state, these opposing forces are essentially equal, and the volume of each component of the ECF remains stable. When the capillary hydrostatic pressure is reduced, such as occurs in hypovolemia, there is increased movement of fluid from the ISF to the IVF. With hypervolemia the reverse situation prevails.

Other substances that do not pass through cell membranes, but which are capable of attracting water (such as glucose), also contribute to the osmotic pressure of the ECF.

Body-fluid Disturbances

Disorders of body-fluid balance can be divided into three general categories: (a) disturbances in osmolality or concentration; (b) disturbances in extracellular fluid volume; and (c) electrolyte and acid-base disturbances.[2] Yet although considered separately, these disturbances are interrelated, and can occur alone or in combination in any individual patient. When the kidneys are functioning normally, the extent of the changes associated with fluid and electrolyte distur-

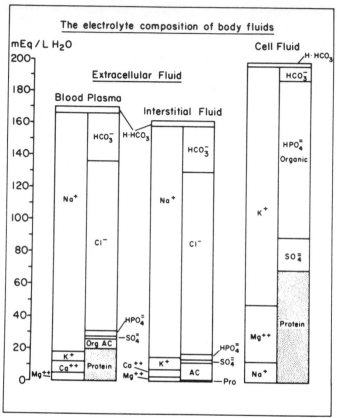

Fig. 1-1.   The electrolyte composition of body fluids (From: Teaching Syllabus for the Course on Fluid and Electrolyte Balance, ed. Scribner BH. Seattle, Washington; University Book Store, 1969. p 4.)

bance can be minimized, particularly if the loss or gain in one or both of these constituents is gradual. A sudden, rapid disturbance in fluid or electrolyte balance overwhelms renal compensatory capabilities, with more severe resulting manifestations. Generally, all losses or gains of fluid and electrolytes occur initially from the ECF.[2]

It is beyond the scope of this chapter to elaborate upon or discuss all of the clinical situations associated with body-fluid disturbances. Numerous other sources deal with these. However, examples of conditions leading to each disturbance will be provided, in an effort to facilitate understanding of the basic pathophysiologic processes underlying each of these specific types of disorder.

DISTURBANCES OF BODY-FLUID OSMOLALITY (CONCENTRATION)

As noted earlier in this chapter, the total concentration of osmotically active particles in the different body-fluid compartments varies from 280 to 295 mOsm/L. If, in either the ECF or the ICF this concentration is singularly altered, water will be redistributed in the direction of the compartment having the greater concentration, until the compartments achieve an equal concentration (isoosmolality), even though the resultant total body osmolality is less or greater than normal. When this happens, the fluid volume of the compartment with the greater particle concentration expands, while the volume of the other compartment contracts.

Since two-thirds of the total body water is located within the cells, changes in water distribution primarily affect cellular volume. Thus, the clinical manifestations of osmolar imbalance result from the shrinkage or swelling of cells.

The osmolality of a body fluid can be measured directly, by the method of freezing point depression, or can be estimated from the serum Na^+ level.[5] Since the osmolality of both the ICF and the ECF must be equal, a measure of the concentration of solutes in either will reflect the concentration in the other.[7] The ECF is easily sampled, and since Na^+ comprises 90 percent of the ECF cation complement (one-half of the ECF osmolality), a measure of the serum Na^+ concentration will reflect total body osmolality. For example, a serum Na^+ of 145 mEq/L, doubled to account for an equal number of anions, reveals an approximate osmolality of 290 mOsm/L, a normal value.

When in the IVF, glucose also exerts an osmotic force, and blood glucose levels should be considered when estimating body osmolality. Hyperglycemia draws water from the cells, diluting the plasma Na^+ concentration. Thus, observation of only the serum Na^+ value under such circumstances would appear to indicate a reduced ECF osmolality when, in fact, the ECF osmolality may be normal or elevated because of the elevated blood glucose.[8] In estimating the influence of blood glucose levels on osmolality, a rough guideline can be used: each 100 mg-percent elevation of blood glucose above normal is approximately equal to a 3 mEq/L rise in serum Na^+.[2]

Hypoosmolar Disturbances (Hyponatremia)

A reduced serum Na^+ concentration (less than 130 mEq/L) indicates a decreased amount of solute, relative to the amount of water, in the body fluid compartments. This hyponatremia is not reflective of total body Na^+ content, since the latter may be high, low, or normal; rather, such hyponatremia reflects the amount of water in which the solutes are dispersed. If, for example, one liter of pure water were to be added (such as by intravenous infusion) to the ECF, the solute concentration of this compartment would decrease, or would be diluted by, the infused water; water would then move into the more concentrated ICF compartment until isoosmolality had been achieved. Thus both the ECF and ICF compartments would share the excess water burden—the ICF compartment to a greater degree because of its larger size—and the overall osmolality of the body would be decreased.

With normally functioning kidneys, a refractory state of hyponatremia is rarely observed.[4] When cells (osmoreceptors) in or near the supraoptic nucleus of the hypothalamus swell in response to an excess of water, the secretion of antidiuretic hormone (ADH) from the pituitary gland is inhibited. In consequence, the renal collecting tubules—the targeted site of ADH action—become less permeable to the resorption of water, and water excretion increases. In addition, swelling of the cells of the lateral preoptic area of the hypothalamus inhibits thirst, so that water intake is curtailed.[3] Both of these mechanisms facilitate the return of water balance to normal.

A reduction in serum Na^+ can develop in persons who have sustained a head injury sufficient to disturb the ADH secretory mechanism; hyponatremia occurs when hypotonic fluids are given to such patients at a time when ADH secretion is excessive.[8] Other potent stimuli for the increased or inappropriate secretion of ADH include a decrease in the effective arterial blood volume, and severe physiologic and psychologic stress.[2,3] A number of other clinical conditions—either alone or in combination with loss or gain of sodium—are also associated with hyponatremia. Examples of these conditions will be considered in the section on combined fluid disorders.

The clinical manifestations of hyponatremia result from cell swelling. Central nervous system (CNS) signs of increased intracranial pressure (ICP) predominate. With a moderate water excess, muscle twitching, hyperreflexia, alterations in behavior, attention, and alertness, and other signs of increased ICP are noted. With severe water intoxication, seizures, coma, hyperventilation, loss of reflexes, and other motor and sensory abnormalities associated with the decompensated phase of increased ICP may occur. Accompanying the CNS signs are increased salivation and lacrimation, watery diarrhea, and "fingerprinting" of the skin.[2,7]

The therapeutic measures employed to correct hyponatremia depend upon the severity of the manifestations of this condition. With moderate water excess, fluid restriction may be all that is necessary. In this way both insensible water losses amount to 600 to 1000 ml per day and obligatory renal water losses can correct the disorder.

When the manifestations of severe hyponatremia are apparent, the administration of hypertonic NaCl solutions (3 to 5 percent) is warranted, though not without danger.[7] By increasing the osmolality of the ECF, these solutions draw water from the cells to the ECF, in which it is available for excretion by the kidneys. A transient increase in ECF volume, from administration of hypertonic saline solutions, may be deleterious to the patient with borderline cardiac compensation. Likewise, changes in ICF volume are associated with harmful neurologic abnormalities.[4] Generally, therefore hypertonic salt solutions should be administered cautiously, with close monitoring of neurologic and cardiovascular status.

Hyperosmolar Disturbances (Hypernatremia)

A serum Na^+ concentration of greater than 150 mEq/L indicates an increase in the solute concentration of body fluids relative to the amount of water present.

A loss of pure water without water replacement will produce an increase in ECF osmolality, a secondary transfer of water from the ICF to the ECF, a reduction in ICF volume, and a generalized state of hyperosmolality.[5]

In response to a hyperosmolar state, the pituitary secretion of ADH increases, with subsequent renal water retention. Thirst receptors are also stimulated and, in combination with ADH, foster a return of water balance to normal. Water loss of sufficient magnitude to reduce ECF volume will stimulate the adrenal release of aldosterone, with a resultant increase in renal Na^+ and water resorption.[9]

In critically ill or debilitated patients with altered levels of consciousness or difficulties in swallowing, hyperosmolality can result from a water intake that is inadequate to replace obligatory insensible and sensible water losses. An impaired sense of thirst, such as may occur in the elderly with cerebral atherosclerosis, or in patients with cerebral disease or injury, can also result in insufficient water intake.[5] Accelerated evaporative lung-water losses may follow hyperventilation associated with fever, cerebral injury, or an unhumidified tracheostomy.[2] A decrease in ADH secretion (central diabetes insipidus), or an inability of the kidneys to respond to the presence of ADH (nephrogenic diabetes insipidus) will lead to renal water wasting and hypernatremia.[4]

Clinically, hypernatremia from pure water loss is manifested by thirst, muscular weakness, and alterations in mentation and orientation. With severe water deficit, delirium, manic behavior, fever, and hypotension may occur; the skin may be flushed, and the mucus membranes may become dry and sticky.[7]

Correction of pure hyperosmolar disturbances requires the administration of free water, either orally or parenterally. However, since rapid restoration of cellular volume can produce potentially harmful water intoxication, the correction of hypernatremia must be accomplished slowly. The extent of water deficit can be calculated from formulas that are available; usually only one-half of the desired volume is replaced in the first 24 hours.[4]

EXTRACELLULAR FLUID VOLUME IMBALANCES

Since Na^+ (with Cl^- and HCO_3^-) comprises the major osmotic element in the movement of water from the ICF to the ECF compartment, the total concentration of Na^+ in the ECF determines the volume of that compartment. Put in another way, the size of the ECF space is an index of total body Na^+ balance.

If Na^+ and water are both lost or gained, and in the same concentrations at which they exist in the plasma (an isotonic change), the osmolar concentration of the ECF does not change, and there is no net transfer of water between the ICF and the ECF. Only the volume of the ECF changes. For example, the loss of a large volume of isotonic gastrointestinal fluid is accompanied by a corresponding reduction in ECF volume. However, since the solute concentration of the fluids lost is the same as that of the remaining fluid, osmolality remains unaffected, and ICF volume remains static.

With the exception of plasma volume measurement no currently available laboratory test can confirm the presence of ECF volume disorders.[2] In some instances of acute ECF loss, an elevated hematocrit may be noted owing to hemoconcentration. The reverse would be true with rapid ECF gain. However, the interpretation of hematocrit in such cases is influenced by recent blood loss or preexisting anemia.

Extracellular Fluid Volume Deficit

Depletion of the ECF volume is associated with a decrease in the total body Na^+ content, and occurs frequently in the critically ill. Gastrointestinal fluid losses resulting from prolonged nasogastric suction, protracted vomiting, diarrhea, or fistula drainage are mainly isotonic or slightly hypotonic in effect, with a marked loss of Na^+, other electrolytes, and water.[2,10] (The electrolyte composition of various gastrointestinal fluids is summarized in Table 1-1). Loss of these fluids results in a contraction of the ECF volume, with little or no change in body osmolality, and thus with minimal change in the ICF volume.

Hemorrhagic shock leads to ECF volume depletion from the external loss of blood and plasma, as well as from a probable internal redistribution of ECF into the cells, particularly skeletal muscle cells.[2]

The sequestration of isotonic ECF into tissue spaces or body cavities (often referred to as "third spacing") results in a reduction in the functional ECF, even though the total ECF volume may be normal or increased.[2] The internal sequestration of ECF is found in cases of burns, peritonitis, intestinal obstruction, extensive soft tissue injury, and hepatic failure.

In response to a reduced plasma volume and to a number of concurrently activated mechanisms, normally functioning kidneys will avidly conserve Na^+ and water. Specific arterial volume receptors, sensitive to changes in plasma volume and renal perfusion, stimulate the secretion of aldosterone through the renin-angiotensin system, enhancing renal Na^+ resorption.[6]

A state of ECF volume depletion is recognized clinically from a number of fairly specific signs and symptoms. Cardiovascular and CNS manifestations are most prominent and depend upon the extent to which the plasma volume has been diminished. With rapid, profound ECF volume depletion, hypotension, cold ashen extremities, distant heart sounds, a subnormal body temperature, and absent peripheral pulses may be evident.[7] Urine volume may be reduced to oliguric levels, and the urine Na^+ content may be negligible. In volume depletion of longer duration, blood urea nitrogen (BUN) levels will rise, reflecting a reduced urea clearance associated with a decreased glomerular filtration rate (GFR).[2] A marked reduction in cerebral perfusion leads to mental confusion, stupor, coma, decreased tendon reflexes, and distal-extremity anesthesia. Nausea, vomiting, paralytic ileus, and sunken eyes may also be noted. Moderate ECF depletion is characterized by less extreme signs and includes postural hypotension, tachycardia, decreased neck vein filling, a collapsing pulse, drowsiness, apathy, and anorexia.[2,7]

The principal medical therapy for significant volume depletion, when unaccompanied by other body fluid disorders, is restoration of the plasma volume by

TABLE 1-1. Water and Electrolyte Losses in Gastrointestinal Secretions and Sweat (After Lockwood, and Randall).

Fluid	Average Volume (ml per 24 hr)	Electrolyte Concentrations (mEq/liter)			
		Na+	K+	Cl-	HCO3-
Blood plasma		136–145	3.5– 5.5	98–106	23–28
Gastric juice[a]	2500				
achlorhydric		8–120	1–30	100	20
containing HCl		10–110	1–32	8– 55	0
Bile	700–1000	134–156	3.9– 6.3	83–110	38
Pancreatic juice	>1000	113–153	2.6– 7.4	54– 95	110
Small bowel (Miller-Abbott suction)	3000	72–120	3.5–6.8	69–127	30
Ileostomy					
(a) recent	100–4000	112–142	4.5–14	93–122	30
(b) adapted	100–500	50	3	20	15–30
Cecostomy	100–3000	48–116	11.1–28.3	35–70	15
Feces	100	<10	<10	<15	<15
Sweat	500–4000	30–70	0– 5	30–70	0

[a]The electrolyte concentrations in gastric juice vary widely—the higher the acidity, the lower the sodium concentration. Thus, when normal gastric acidity is present, the average sodium concentration of gastric juice is approximately 45 mEq/L. When hypoacidity or anacidity is present (as in elderly patients or those with carcinoma of the stomach), the average sodium concentration of gastric juice is approximately 100 mEq/L. (From: Goldberger E: A Primer of Water, Electrolyte and Acid–Base Syndromes, 6th edn. Philadelphia, Lea and Febiger, 1980. pp 77.)

infusion of a balanced salt solution, such as lactated Ringer's solution.[10] The adequacy of fluid replacement therapy toward achieving hemodynamic stability can be determined by frequent assessment of heart rate, blood pressure, urine output, and cerebral function. However, in the critically ill patient with complex fluid disorders, these traditional indices may be insufficient to accurately establish the volume status.[11] In such instances, more sophisticated and invasive monitoring of hemodynamic variables is necessary. (See Chapter 3 for a further discussion of these techniques.)

Extracellular Fluid Volume Excess

An ECF overload is associated with an excess of total body Na+ and is manifested primarily by edema. Pathophysiologically, addition of isotonic fluid to the ECF, without corresponding ECF loss, results in a circulatory and interstitial volume expansion, with minimal changes in osmolality or ICF volume.

The majority of cases of ECF volume overload are either iatrogenic or due to inappropriate renal retention of water.[10] Overinfusion of Na+-containing fluids or plasma expanders, or the administration of salt solutions to patients in oliguric renal failure, rapidly results in circulatory overload. In the elderly or in patients with marginal cardiac reserve, moderate volume excess may lead to acute congestive heart failure and pulmonary edema.

An increase in circulating aldosterone is a potent stimulus for continued Na+ and water resorption in the distal convoluting tubule. Enhancement of aldosterone secretion results from factors that decrease effective arterial blood volume (such as hemorrhage or Na^+ depletion), from hyperkalemia, and from increased adrenocorticotrophic hormone levels.[7]

Weight gain is often the earliest sign of a developing ECF volume excess. Unless adequate nutrition is maintained in critically ill patients who are catabolic, weight losses may range from one-fourth to one-half pound per day. During a catabolic period, a stable weight or a weight gain in the absence of nutritional support may indicate retention of ECF in these patients. Distended peripheral veins, increased cardiac output, a bounding pulse, and peripheral edema also may appear.

The treatment of ECF volume excess depends upon the physiologic mechanisms responsible for its development. General measures that may be used to reduce volume overload include restriction of Na^+-containing foods, fluids, or medications; administration of diuretics; and peritoneal or hemodialysis. In addition, efforts toward improvement of cardiac, renal, and hepatic function are also undertaken.

COMBINED OSMOLAR AND VOLUME DISORDERS

The coexistence of osmolar and volume imbalances is not unusual in severely ill persons. The recognition of these mixed disorders is made easier if the distinguishing features of each component are considered separately. An additive effect may occur when the signs of both osmolar and volume imbalance are alike. Opposite signs tend to cancel each other.[2]

In instances in which lost large volumes of isotonic fluid are replaced with hypotonic fluids, or in which hypotonic fluid losses occur without fluid intake, ECF volume depletion and hyponatremia can develop. The addition of hypotonic fluids to a depleted ECF compartment will only slightly expand the ECF volume, reduce the ECF osmolality, cause a net movement of water into the ICF compartment, and will thus expand the ICF volume. The ECF deficit will then coexist with a hypoosmolar imbalance.

ECF volume overload and hypernatremia can be produced by the excessive administration of salt solutions during periods of water restriction, by the replacement of pure-water losses with Na^+-containing solutions, or by the excessive administration of hypertonic agents (such as $NaHCO_3^-$, glucose, or mannitol).[7] The addition of $NaHCO_3^-$ to the ECF increases the ECF osmolality, causing a shift of water from the ICF to the ECF compartment. The ECF volume thus expands, while the ICF volume contracts, and the overall osmolality is elevated. Hyponatremia and ECF volume excess can occur when hypotonic fluids or water are given to persons in renal failure.

The therapeutic approach to correction of mixed fluid disorders is determined, in part, by the severity of patient manifestations, and entails combining of the corrective measures for each individual disorder. Restoration or preservation of normal renal function will ease the correction of imbalances by permitting the ready excretion of excess solute and water.

POTASSIUM IMBALANCES

All but approximately 2 percent of the total body K^+ is located in the intracellular water, at a concentration of 150 mEq/L. The ECF K^+ concentration is normally between 4 and 5 mEq/L.[12] These levels must be maintained within very narrow limits to ensure a critical level of cardiac and neuromuscular function.

Potassium balance depends primarily upon the regulation of K^+ excretion by the kidneys. Since K^+ is ubiquitous in natural foods, renal mechanisms normally favor K^+ excretion; wide variations in daily K^+ intake evoke immediate and corresponding adjustments in renal K^+ excretion.

The rate at which K^+ is excreted is determined by the concentration of K^+ in the distal tubular cells. A high cellular K^+ concentration is associated with a more rapid K^+ excretion and vice versa.[12] On the other hand, the concentration of K^+ in the urine depends upon the amount of Na^+ delivered to the distal tubules for resorption, on the amount of K^+ secreted into the tubular lumen, on the degree of urine acidification, and on the level of adrenocorticotrophic hormone (ACTH). Thus, during diuretic therapy (as with furosemide, ethacrynic acid, or thiazides,), or with an osmotic diuresis, greater amounts of Na^+ are delivered to the distal tubule where, under the influence of aldosterone, this Na^+ is resorbed while K^+ is excreted. Rapid or prolonged administration of potassium-free NaCl solutions induces a kaliuresis by this same mechanism.[12]

The distribution of K^+ between the ICF and the ECF is influenced by several factors. Both aldosterone and insulin have been recognized to control the cellular uptake of K^+.[12] Acidosis causes a shift of intracellular K^+ to the ECF, while alkalosis results in an opposite shift. Severe physiologic stress and catabolic states can release significant quantities of intracellular K^+ into the ECF.

The serum K^+ level, in the absence of acid–base imbalances or other causes of distributional K^+ changes, is used as an indication of total body K^+ stores. According to rough estimates, a decrease in the normal serum K^+ of 1 mEq/L corresponds to a loss of about 200 to 300 mEq of K^+ from body stores. Similar information is not available for K^+ excess.[12]

Hypokalemia

Mechanisms of K^+ depletion include decreased potassium intake, increased renal potassium excretion, and excessive extrarenal potassium loss. An internal shift of K^+ into cells results in hypokalemia followed by an increase in renal K^+ excretion.

Symptomatic K^+ depletion resulting solely from dietary deprivation is infrequent other than in the very ill who are kept on a low intake for long periods.[12] The loss of upper gastrointestinal fluids through vomiting or suction can result in K^+ depletion, primarily through increased renal excretion, since these fluids contain relatively small amounts of K^+.[13] The mechanism by which K^+ depletion occurs from loss of upper gastrointestinal fluid is as follows: Loss of gastric hydrochloric acid and Na^+ results in a metabolic alkalosis and ECF volume depletion; K^+ shifts into the cells in exchange for H^+, producing hypokalemia. In the kidney, HCO_3^- and Na^+ are presented to the distal tubules in large amounts. Na^+ and Cl^- are preferentially resorbed in exchange for K^+ and HCO_3^-, which are excreted. If the Cl^- depletion in this instance is not corrected, the metabolic alkalosis will be maintained. The continued demand for Na^+ conservation, without adequate Cl^- anion to be resorbed with this Na^+, produces HCO_3^- resorption, with continued K^+ and H^+ excretion. The resulting depletion of K^+ evokes a greater excretion of H^+ and a further perpetuation of the metabolic alkalosis.

Lower intestinal fluids have a high K^+ content, and loss of these results in K^+ depletion. In edema-forming states such as congestive heart failure, nephrotic syndrome, and hepatic cirrhosis, K^+ loss occurs because of metabolic alkalosis, diuretic therapy, and increased levels of circulating aldosterone.

With moderate K^+ depletion, outward clinical signs may be absent. Clinical manifestations in cases of larger K^+ deficit result from alterations in transmembrane potential and the excitability of neuromuscular tissues. Muscle weakness occurs early and can proceed to generalized areflexia, paralysis, and death from respiratory muscle failure.[2] Degenerative changes in muscle tissue may progress, in severe K^+ depletion, to frank rhabdomyolysis and myoglobinuria.[12]

Cardiac abnormalities of K^+ depletion include bradycardia, supraventricular and ventricular arrhythmias, and alterations in conduction. A depressed ST segment, flattened T wave, and increased U wave voltage may be seen in the electrocardiogram (ECG). Digitalis toxicity is exaggerated by K^+ depletion. Metabolically, there develops in K^+ depletion states a glucose intolerance that results partially from impaired insulin release and partially from a defect in peripheral glucose utilization.[13] An important renal effect of K^+ depletion is a decrease in tubular concentrating ability, leading to polyuria, nocturia, and polydipsia.

The primary goals of therapy for K^+ depletion are correction of the K^+ deficit and prevention of further imbalances. As a general rule, K^+ deficits that are corrected through intravenous therapy are corrected slowly, so as to avoid the development of transient but dangerous hyperkalemia. Usually, no greater than 20 mEq/L or 100 to 150 mEq/day of K^+ should be administered, unless the patient's K^+ deficit is life-threatening.[2] When more rapid replacements are indicated, ECG monitoring and frequent measurement of serum K^+ levels are essential. Oral K^+ supplements are preferred, if possible, because the gradual rate of gastrointestinal K^+ absorption with these lessens the chance for hyperkalemia. Since the major route of K^+ excretion is renal, adequate kidney function must be insured during the administration of K^+ supplements.

Hyperkalemia

The development of K^+ excess and hyperkalemia can result from an impairment of renal excretory function, from a movement of intracellular K^+ into the ECF, or from an iatrogenic overdose of K^+ supplement to patients with renal insufficiency. Oliguric renal failure, hypoaldosteronism, or the use of K^+-sparing diuretics decreases the ability of the kidneys to excrete K^+. Rapid cell break-down, such as is associated with major trauma, crush injuries, or burns, can release large amounts of K^+ into the ECF. Metabolic acidosis causes a shift of intracellular K^+ to the ECF, and with a resultant increase in serum K^+ levels.

As with hypokalemia, the clinical manifestations of hyperkalemia result from an electrophysiologic disturbance in muscular function. There may be muscle weakness progressing to flaccid paralysis. Cardiac toxicity is manifested early in the ECG in the form of symmetrical peaking of T waves, widening of the QRS complex, and lengthening of the PR interval. With more severe hyper-kalemia, heart block, a disappearance of the P wave, and a merging of the QRS and T wave into a sine wave pattern occurs. Ventricular fibrillation and asystole closely follow upon the appearance of the sine wave pattern.[12]

The method used for reducing serum K^+ levels depends upon the severity of the toxic effects of the hyperkalemia and the rapidity with which the patient's serum K^+ levels have risen. Temporary reversal of cardiac depression can be accomplished by intravenous administration of calcium gluconate, which re-stores resting membrane postential; Na^+ lactate or $NaHCO_3^-$, which raise the pH of the ECF and facilitate the transfer of K^+ into the cells; or glucose and insulin, which enhance cellular K^+ uptake.[12] However, since these measures are only temporarily useful, more definitive measures to remove excess K^+ from the body are necessary. In cases of obvious cardiotoxicity and in which renal function cannot be restored, peritoneal or hemodialysis may be instituted. In cases with more slowly increasing serum K^+ levels, cation exchange resins, given orally or rectally, can control serum K^+ levels. In milder hyperkalemic states, restriction of exogenous K^+ intake may suffice to correct the problem.

CALCIUM IMBALANCES

Most of the body's calcium (Ca^{2+}) is found in the skeleton. The remainder is in the ECF, and accounts for a normal serum Ca^{2+} concentration of 9 to 11 mg percent.[14] The major portion of daily ingested Ca^{2+} is excreted in the feces, and a lesser portion is excreted by kidneys.

The total serum Ca^{2+} concentration is a summed measure of three compo-nents: Ca^{2+} bound to protein—mainly to albumin; Ca^{2+} complexed with other substances, such as phosphate; and ionized Ca^{2+}. Approximately 50 percent of the total serum Ca^{2+} is in ionized form, and it is this portion that is responsible for regulating neuromuscular function.

In order to analyze the ionized Ca^{2+} concentration when direct measure-ment techniques are unavailable, a determination of plasma protein levels is important[15]; the level of protein-bound Ca^{2+} will determine the ratio of ionized Ca^{2+} in the serum. The ionized Ca^{2+} concentration can be estimated from the rough rule that each gram of serum albumin binds approximately 0.9 mg of Ca^{2+}.[16] Nomograms for this purpose are also available.

Blood pH changes affect the Ca^{2+}-binding capacity of plasma protein and, therefore, influence ionized Ca^{2+} concentrations. Alkalosis reduces ionized Ca^{2+}

by enhancing protein binding; conversely, acidosis increases ionized Ca^{2+} levels.[2]

A stable serum Ca^{2+} concentration normally depends upon an interaction of several regulatory mechanisms: parathyroid hormone (PTH), calcitonin, and vitamin D.[14] PTH is responsible for raising depressed serum Ca^{2+} levels, whereas calcitonin lowers serum Ca^{2+} levels. Disturbances in Ca^{2+} balance result from alterations in these regulatory mechanisms, in bone metabolism, or in Ca^{2+} intake.

Hypocalcemia

The reduction in serum Ca^{2+} observed in acute or chronic renal failure is a result of renal phosphate retention, reduced renal activation of vitamin D, decreased intestinal Ca^{2+} absorption, and impaired skeletal response to PTH. Other causes of hypocalcemia include hypoparathyroidism, magnesium deficiency, acute pancreatitis, and massive soft-tissue infection.[2, 17]

An increase in neuromuscular irritability, producing tetany, is the basis of the clinical manifestations of hypocalcemia. Numbness and tingling of the fingers, toes, and circumoral region, carpopedal spasms, hyperactive reflexes, a positive Chvostek's sign, and prolongation of the QT interval on the ECG may appear. Seizures can accompany severe Ca^{2+} deficits.[14,16]

Repletion of Ca^{2+} deficits occurs simultaneously with measures directed at correcting the underlying cause of the disorder responsible for such deficits. Calcium gluconate or calcium chloride may be cautiously administered to correct acute symptoms of hypocalcemia. Oral Ca^{2+} and vitamin D supplements may be administered when more chronic therapy is indicated.

Hypercalcemia

Metastatic or primary bone neoplasias and hyperparathyroidism are the two most common causes of hypercalcemia in hospitalized patients.[16] An augmentation of high serum calcium levels found in these conditions can result from concomitant ECF volume depletion or prolonged periods of immobility with bone demineralization. In patients undergoing treatment for chronic renal failure, an elevated serum Ca^{2+} can be attributed to factors such as secondary hyperparathyroidism, excessive vitamin D or C^{2+} intake, phosphate depletion, or high concentration of Ca^{2+} in dialysates.[16, 17]

The clinical manifestations of hypercalcemia involve the renal, musculoskeletal, gastrointestinal, cardiovascular, and central nervous systems. These manifestations include nephrolithiasis, azotemia, and decreased renal concentrating ability; varying degrees of muscular weakness, apathy, and decreasing mental alertness; nausea and vomiting; anorexia, vague abdominal pains, and paralytic ileus; hypertension, and shortening of the QT interval with later widening of the T wave on the ECG.[2,16]

The management of hypercalcemia includes general supportive measures to impede further increases in serum Ca^{2+} and the resultant complications of this, measures to lower the serum Ca^{2+} concentration, and measures to correct the underlying cause of the hypercalcemia. Important general measures include replenishment of ECF volume deficits to facilitate Ca^{2+} excretion, correction of existing electrolyte abnormalities, increasing patient mobility, and discontinuation or adjustment of medications that raise serum Ca^{2+}.

Potent diuretics such as furasemide (Lasix) or ethycrinic acid (Edecrin), and sodium chloride or sodium sulfate infusions, enhance urinary Ca^{2+} losses. Hemodialysis reduces hypercalcemia in patients with inadequate renal function. Inhibition of bone resorption can be achieved through the administration of calcitonin, although the effect of this is limited, and by the administration of intravenous mithramycin, an antineoplastic agent. Inorganic phosphates lower serum Ca^{2+} levels by augmenting the rate of bone deposition. Intravenous infusion of these latter substances must be regulated carefully so as to avoid precipitous decreases in the serum Ca^{2+} level, and extraskeletal calcifications.[16]

MAGNESIUM IMBALANCES

As the second most abundant intracellular cation, Mg^{2+} plays a major role in activating multiple essential enzyme systems necessary for cellular function. Mg^{2+}-dependent ATP synthesis is vital for the maintenance of intracellular Na^+-K^+ pumps, muscular contraction, and carbohydrate utilization.[10]

Serum Mg^{2+} levels, which normally range from 1.6 to 2.1 mEq/L, are useful in screening patients with suspected magnesium imbalances. However, the serum Mg^{2+} concentration is often an unreliable indicator of total Mg^{2+} stores.[18]

Magnesium Deficit

Vulnerability to Mg^{2+} depletion is notable in chronic alcoholic patients, who, because of inadequate nutrient intake, vomiting, diarrhea, and increased renal excretion lose significant quantities of Mg^{2+}. Patients undergoing long-term parenteral therapy without Mg^{2+} supplements and prolonged gastric suction also can develop Mg^{2+} deficits.[15]

Tetany characterizes the clinical picture of Mg^{2+} deficiency. The signs and symptoms of the deficiency are very similar to those of hypocalcemia. The symptoms of Mg^{2+} deficit are potentiated by hypocalcemia, and these two disorders have frequently been found to coexist.[18]

Magnesium sulfate solutions can be administered parenterally to correct existing Mg^{2+} deficits, although caution must be exercised in order to avoid adverse cardiac effects induced by sudden hypermagnesemia.

Magnesium Excess

Cases of Mg^{2+} excess are most frequently encountered clinically in patients with renal failure who ingest large doses of Mg^{2+}-containing antacids or laxatives. In addition, massive tissue destruction or cell catabolism, such as occurs with trauma or diabetic ketoacidosis, can release intracellular Mg^{2+} into the ECF, producing hypermagnesemia.

Signs and symptoms of Mg^{2+} excess resemble those of hyperkalemia, and result from the impedance of neuromuscular transmission and depression of cardiac contractility.[15]

In patients with normal renal function, cessation of exogenous sources of Mg^{2+} is often sufficient to correct Mg^{2+} excess. Severe neuromuscular and cardiac symptoms can be temporarily controlled through the administration of Ca^{2+}, which antagonizes the action of Mg^{2+}, or by glucose and insulin, which enhance the intracellular movement of Mg^{2+}. In patients with renal failure, hemodialysis provides an effective rapid means for removing Mg^{2+} from the body.[18]

ACID–BASE DISORDERS

Acid–base balance in the body depends upon the maintenance of a fixed ratio of acidic to basic substances in the body fluids. This ratio is defined by the Henderson-Hasselbalch equation, which discloses that as long as the concentration of base to acid is 20:1—no matter what the absolute values of either—the pH of the body fluid will remain at an average normal value of 7.4.[19] The pH is a measure of the hydrogen ion (H^+) concentration of body fluids; the body has an extremely efficient control system for preserving this ratio.

The daily acid load produced by the metabolism of food substrates is rapidly neutralized by a number of buffer systems, and the resultant products are finally excreted by the lungs and kidneys. Buffer systems consist of paired chemicals: a weakly ionized acid or base and the fully ionized salt of that acid or base. Buffers accomplish their task by binding or releasing H^+ in response to changes in H^+ concentration.

In the ECF, constancy of the H^+ concentration is maintained principally by the bicarbonate–carbonic acid ($HCO_3^- - H_2CO_3$) buffer system; other ECF buffers, namely hemoglobin, phosphate ions, and plasma protein, provide additional acid neutralization but to a lesser extent. Important intracellular buffers include organic phosphates, protein, and bicarbonate.

When a metabolic acid enters the ECF it ionizes, and H^+ derived from the acid combines with HCO_3^- to form H_2CO_3 and a salt of the acid. The H_2CO_3 is rapidly converted to carbon dioxide (CO_2) and water, both of which are excreted by the lungs. H^+ arising from acids other than H_2CO_3 (such as sulfuric or phosphoric acid) must be excreted by the kidneys.[20] Disturbances in either pulmonary or renal function can result in significant derangements of body acid–base balance.

There are four types of acid–base disturbance[2]; these are summarized in Table 1-2. The acid–base status of patients is determined by an analysis of arterial blood gases. The arterial pH establishes body acidity or alkalinity, while the pCO_2 reflects the contribution of the pulmonary system to the acid–base disturbance; the standard HCO_3^- defines the metabolic contribution to such a

TABLE 1-2. Acidosis–Alkalosis

Type of Acid–Base Disorder	Defect	Common Causes	$\dfrac{BHCO_3}{H_2CO_3} = \dfrac{20}{1}$	Compensation
Respiratory acidosis	Retention of CO_2 (decreased alveolar ventilation)	Depression of respiratory center—morphine, CNS injury Pulmonary disease—emphysema, pneumonia	↑ Denominator Ratio less than 20:1	Renal Retention of bicarbonate, excretion of acid salts, increased ammonia formation Chloride shift into red cells
Respiratory alkalosis	Excessive loss of CO_2 (increased alveolar ventilation)	Hyperventilation: Emotional, severe pain, assisted ventilation, encephalitis	↓ Denominator Ratio greater than 20:1	Renal Excretion of bicarbonate, retention of acid salts, decreased ammonia formation
Metabolic acidosis	Retention of fixed acids or loss of base bicarbonate	Diabetes, azotemia, lactic acid accumulation, starvation Diarrhea, small bowel fistulae	↓ Numerator Ratio less than 20:1	Pulmonary (rapid) Increase rate and depth of breathing Renal (slow) As in respiratory acidosis
Metabolic alkalosis	Loss of fixed acids Gain of base bicarbonate Potassium depletion	Vomiting or gastric suction with pyloric obstruction Excessive intake of bicarbonate Diuretics	↑ Numerator Ratio greater than 20:1	Pulmonary (rapid) Decrease rate and depth of breathing Renal (slow) As in respiratory alkalosis

From: Shires GT, Canizaro PC: Fluid, electrolyte, and nutritional management of the surgical patient. In: Principles of Surgery, 3rd edn., eds. Schwartz SI, et al. New York, McGraw-Hill, 1979. pp 71.

disturbance. In complicated acid–base disorders, it is often difficult to establish whether changes in pCO_2 or HCO_3^- represent coexisting primary disorders or compensatory responses to a primary acid–base disorder. In such instances, determination of base excess or base deficit—the amount of strong acid or base per liter of blood—is useful in separating and quantifying the metabolic component of the acid–base disturbance.[7]

The treatment of acid–base disturbances includes correction of the underlying clinical derangement responsible for the disturbance, and correction of associated fluid and electrolyte imbalances. For cases in which acidosis is so severe as to threaten life (such as those with a pH below 7.2), partial correction of the pH, by the administration of $NaHCO_3$,[2] is advocated.

REFERENCES

1. Hays RM: Dynamics of body water and electrolytes. In: Clinical Disorders of Fluid and Electrolyte Metabolism, 3rd edn. eds. Maxwell MH and Kleeman CR. New York; McGraw-Hill, 1980, pp 1–36
2. Shires GT, Canizaro PC: Fluid, electrolyte, and nutritional management of the surgical patient. In: Principles of Surgery, 3rd edn., eds. Schwartz SI et al. New York; McGraw-Hill, 1979, pp 65–97
3. Ramsay DJ, Ganong WF: CNS regulation of salt and water intake. Hospital Practice, 12(3):63–69, 1977
4. Humes DH, Narins R, Brenner B: Disorders of water balance. Hospital Practice, 14(3):133–145, 1979
5. Burke MD: Electrolyte studies: 1. Sodium and water. Postgrad Med, 64(4):147–153, 1978
6. Levy M: The pathophysiology of sodium balance. Hospital Practice, 13(11):95–106, 1978
7. Goldberger E: A Primer of Water, Electrolyte and Acid–Base Syndromes, 6th edn. Philadelphia; Lea and Febiger, 1980
8. Levin M: Hyponatremic syndromes. Med Clin North Am, 62(6):1257–1272, 1978
9. Klahr S, Slatopolsky E: Renal regulation of sodium excretion: Function in health and edema forming states. Arch Intern Med, 131:780–790, 1973
10. Trunkey D: Review of current concepts in fluid and electrolyte management. Heart and Lung, 4(1):115–121, 1975
11. Horovitz J: Monitoring the injured patient. Bull NY Acad Med, 55(2):163–173, 1979
12. Cohen J: The kidney in health and disease: VII: Disorders of potassium balance, Hospital Practice, 14(1):119–128, 1979
13. Zeluff G, Suki W, Jackson D: Grand rounds in critical care: Hypokalemia—cause and treatment. Heart and Lung, 7(5):854–860, 1978
14. O'Dorisio TM: Hypercalcemic crisis. Heart and Lung, 7(3):425–434, 1978
15. Parfitt AM, Kleerekoper M: Clinical disorders of calcium, phosphorus, and magnesium metabolism. In: Clinical Disorders of Fluid and Electrolyte Metabolism, 3rd edn., eds. Maxwell MH, Kleeman CR. New York, McGraw-Hill, 1980. pp 947–1151
16. Lee D, Zawada E, Kleeman C: The pathophysiology and clinical aspects of hypercalcemic disorders. West J Med, 129(4):278–320, 1978
17. Bell NH: Hypercalcemic and hypocalcemic disorders: Diagnosis and treatment. Nephron, 23:147–151, 1979

18. Geiderman JM, Goodman SL, Cohen DB: Magnesium—The forgotten electrolyte. J Am Coll Emerg Phys, 8(5):204–208, 1979
19. Wilson RF, Sibbold WJ: Approach to acid–base problems in the critically ill and injured. J Am Coll Emerg Phys, 5(7):515–522, 1976
20. Quintanilla AP: Acid–base disorders: 1. Laboratory characterization. Postgrad Med, 60(5):68–70, 1976

2 | Functional Hematology

Maribel J. Clements

Blood, which makes up only 8 percent of the total body weight, provides the means for the respiration and nutrition necessary for all body activities. Additionally, some blood constituents control infection and others provide hemostatis.

Nurses, particularly those caring for critically ill patients, must understand the functions of blood and the indications for blood and blood component transfusions. This chapter summarizes the production and function of blood constituents with particular emphasis on red blood cells. Immunohematology and the separation of blood into its components are also briefly reviewed.

COMPOSITION OF BLOOD

Blood is a fluid containing cells in suspension and various chemicals in solution. The average volume of blood in a normal adult is 6 liters but this amount varies with the size of the individual. The blood volume of the body (in milliliters) can be roughly calculated by multiplying a patient's weight in kilograms by 70.

The formed elements of blood including red blood cells (erythrocytes), white blood cells (leukocytes), and platelets (thrombocytes) account for approximately 45 percent of the blood volume. Erythrocytes constitute the majority of these cells. In each cubic millimeter of blood there are normally 4.2 to 6.2 million red cells, 150,000 to 400,000 platelets, and 5,000 to 10,000 leukocytes. Red cells and platelets remain in the blood vessels throughout their life span, but for leukocytes, which are mainly found extravascularly, the blood stream is only a transport system.

There are several different types of leukocytes. Since the proportion of these different types may change in certain disease states, it is important to know the normal values. In a patient with a normal white cell differential count,

21

neutrophils account for approximately 60 percent and lymphocytes for approximately 34 percent of all leukocytes; monocytes, eosinophils, and basophils comprise the remaining 6 percent.

Fifty-five percent of the blood volume is plasma. Plasma is composed of 91.5 percent water and 7 percent protein. The remaining 1.5 percent is made up of inorganic salts, lipids, enzymes, hormones, vitamins, and carbohydrates.

HEMATOPOIESIS

Erythrocytes, leukocytes, and platelets all originate from the same precursor or stem cell. Hematopoiesis is the process by which the cells differentiate, proliferate, mature, and reach the circulating blood. Most of this cell production takes place in the bone marrow, but the liver, spleen, and lymph nodes are also involved.[1]

Erythrocytes

It takes from 5 to 7 days for erythrocytes to reach maturity; their average lifespan in the circulation is 120 days. Erythrocytes are produced in the bone marrow, liver, and spleen. The rate at which reticulocytes (young erythrocytes) are released into the blood stream is determined by the rate at which oxygen is transported to body tissues. A decreased oxygen tension at the tissue level causes an increase in the number of reticulocytes released. Acute anemia due to blood loss is an example of a condition that decreases oxygen tension.

Leukocytes

Leukopoiesis is the development of leukocytes, and it involves the granulocytic series (neutrophils, basophils, and eosinophils) and the nongranulocytic series (lymphocytes and monocytes). The bone-marrow granulocyte pool contains approximately 30 cells for each cell found in circulation; during an infection; the increased number of granulocytes released into the circulation comes from these bone-marrow reserves. The lifespan of the granulocyte is short and thus if there arises a great need for granulocytes, the bone marrow pool can be depleted rapidly unless the rate of granulocyte production is increased. Apparently, specific hormones stimulate granulocyte immature cells in the proliferating bone marrow pool to increase their rate of mitosis, and therefore the rate of granulocyte production.[2]

The bone marrow is a secondary production site of the nongranulocytic leukocyte series; lymphocytes are produced primarily in lymphatic tissue located in the lymph glands, thymus, spleen, and gastrointestinal tract. The major site of monocyte production is unknown.[2]

Platelets

Blood platelets are cell fragments devoid of a nucleus; they are derived from the cytoplasm of the bone marrow cells known as megakaryocytes. The lifespan of platelets in the circulation is approximately 10 days.

CHARACTERISTICS AND FUNCTIONS OF ERYTHROCYTES

The developing erythrocyte in the bone marrow has a nucleus and is capable of mitosis. It can also synthesize DNA, RNA, lipid, protein, and heme. When the immature erythrocyte is released into the blood stream, it is called a reticulocyte; the reticulocyte no longer has a nucleus, and cannot synthesize DNA and RNA.

Approximately 48 hours after entering the blood stream, the reticulocyte becomes a mature erythrocyte. This mature cell depends almost entirely on glucose as its energy source, using anaerobic glycolysis (the Embden-Meyerhof pathway) and the pentose-phosphate pathway for carbohydrate metabolism. The Embden-Meyerhof pathway is normally responsible for 90 percent of the glucose metabolism of the erythrocyte, and produces adenosine triphosphate (ATP) as a metabolic byproduct. ATP, which contains high-energy phosphate bonds, is needed to maintain the integrity of the corpuscular membrane of the erythrocyte, as well as to sustain such energy-requiring processes as the ion-exchange pumps that maintain proper cation concentrations within the cell.[2,3]

A side reaction of the Embden-Meyerhof pathway is the 2,3-diphosphoglycerate (2,3-DPG) shunt. This shunt does not produce energy, and in fact results in decreased energy production when it is in operation. However, the 2,3-DPG produced by the shunt is very important in modulating the amount of oxygen released by hemoglobin to the tissues.[2]

The major function of the erythrocyte is oxygen transport. Hemoglobin, which is contained within the erythrocyte, transports oxygen from the lungs to the tissues, facilitates the removal of carbon dioxide from the tissues, and acts as one of the most important buffers in the blood.

Hemoglobin is produced through the combination of specific polypeptides known as globins, and an iron-containing porphyrin known as heme. Abnormal hemoglobins result from a defect in the globin part of the molecule.

Oxygen Transport

Each hemoglobin molecule contains four oxygen binding sites and transports oxygen by combining with the oxygen molecule. The affinity of hemoglobin for oxygen varies under different physiologic conditions.[4] It was originally thought that the amount of oxygen available to the tissues depended upon the oxygen carrying capacity (the hemoglobin content) of the blood, the oxygen saturation of arterial blood, and the cardiac output. However, not all of the oxygen bound to hemoglobin is readily available to the tissues.

An understanding of the variable affinity of hemoglobin for oxygen, and of the factors that affect this affinity, is important in critical care nursing. Figure 2-1 shows the oxygen–hemoglobin dissociation curve. The oxygen tension or partial pressure of oxygen in the lungs is approximately 100 mmHg. The partial pressure of oxygen in the venous blood is approximately 35 mmHg. The shape of the dissociation curve indicates that the percentage of hemoglobin saturated with oxygen is not directly proportional to the amount of oxygen in the blood. In other words, deoxyhemoglobin (hemoglobin with no oxygen attached) apparently does not take up the first oxygen molecule as readily as it takes up subsequent molecules. In fact, the affinity of hemoglobin for oxygen increases with each oxygen molecule that is added to the hemoglobin molecule, until the latter is saturated with four oxygens. Conversely, the loss of one oxygen lowers the oxygen affinity of the remaining heme groups within the hemoglobin molecule.[5]

The progressive increase in the affinity of hemoglobin for oxygen arises from a structural change in the hemoglobin molecule that permits it to bind oxygen more readily. This change in structure may take place after one, two, or three oxygen molecules have been bound but becomes more probable with each successive oxygen molecule that is bound. The transition in the structures is influenced by hydrogen ions, carbon dioxide, and 2,3-DPG. The higher the concentrations of these substances, the lower the affinity of hemoglobin for oxygen, and vice versa.[5]

Carbon Dioxide Transport

Carbon dioxide released by the tissues is too insoluble to be transported as such. Some of this carbon dioxide binds to hemoglobin, but most of it is transported in the form of biocarbonate ions. For every four oxygen molecules that hemoglobin gives up, it takes up two hydrogen ions. This reciprocal action, known as the Bohr effect, is the key mechanism in carbon dioxide transport. The hemoglobin takes up the hydrogen ions that are produced when carbon dioxide combines with water to form a bicarbonate ion and a hydrogen ion. The chemical reaction for this is

$$CO_2 + H_2O \rightleftharpoons H_2CO_3 \rightleftharpoons HCO_3^- + H^+$$

By taking up these hydrogen ions, hemoglobin permits more carbon dioxide, which is insoluble, to form the bicarbonate ion, which is soluble and which can then be transported to the lungs. When the blood reaches the lungs, oxygen binds to the hemoglobin and the latter casts off the hydrogen ions. The cast-off hydrogen ions combine with bicarbonate ions in the blood to form carbon dioxide and water. The carbon dioxide then diffuses into the alveoli, and is exhaled.[5]

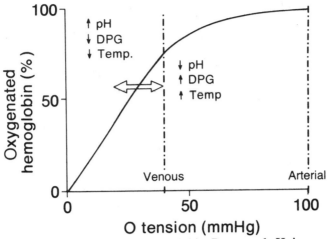

Fig. 2-1.   Oxygen dissociation curve of hemoglobin. Decreased pH, increased 2,3-DPG, and increased temperature shift the curve to the right, making oxygen more readily available to the tissues.

Buffer Action

Oxidation in the tissues liberates lactic and carbonic acids. These acids in turn liberate hydrogen ions. Hemoglobin acts as a buffer by taking up these hydrogen ions.

CHARACTERISTICS AND FUNCTIONS OF LEUKOCYTES

Leukocytes are larger than erythrocytes and retain their nuclei. Cells of the granulocytic leukocyte series are distinguished by having granules in their cytoplasm, and include neutrophils, basophils, and eosinophils. The major role of neutrophils is the phagocytosis, killing, and digestion of microorganisms. The neutrophil usually degenerates after digesting phagocytized bacteria.[6,7]

There are very few basophils in the peripheral blood. These cells contain histamine and are probably associated with acute allergic responses.[6]

Eosinophils, like neutrophils, can ingest and destroy microorganisms. However, it is doubtful that this is their major function, since their numbers in the blood are reduced rather than increased in most infections. Recent evidence suggests that eosinophils play a specific role in defending against certain parasitic infections such as trichinosis. Eosinophils also seem to be involved in modulating the functions of basophils in certain allergic or hypersensitivity diseases.[7]

The nongranulocytic leukocyte series includes lymphocytes and monocytes. There are at least two different types of lymphocytes, T cells and B cells. T cells comprise roughly 70 percent of the lymphocytes in the blood. The major function of these cells is the expression of cellular immunity. When T cells are stimulated, they proliferate and differentiate into cells having specific, active roles in the immune response. These roles range from activities against specific cells or antigens to activities that regulate B-cell responses.

B cells comprise approximately 25 percent of the lymphocytes in the blood. When B cells are stimulated by specific antigens, they produce immunoglobulins (antibodies).[7] These mature B cells are sometimes called plasma cells.

Monocytes are large, slow-moving cells that provide a general purpose cleanup. They share with neutrophils the capacity to engulf and kill bacteria, but they also phagocytize debris.[7]

PRODUCTION AND FUNCTION OF MAJOR PLASMA PROTEINS

The major plasma proteins are albumin, other transport proteins, immunoglobulins, complement components, clotting proteins, and hormones.

Albumin is synthesized in the liver, and constitutes 55 percent of the plasma protein. Albumin is a transport medium for anions, cations, fatty acids, certain hormones, and drugs. Since capillary walls are normally impermeable to albumin, this plasma protein helps to maintain oncotic pressure. Albumin also acts as a buffer.

The level of albumin in the plasma normally remains quite constant, the liver taking up or releasing this protein as needed. In dehydration, intravascular fluid loss causes an increase in the concentration of albumin in the blood. Decreases in body albumin occur with malnutrition, protein-losing gastroenteropathies, nephrotic syndrome, or hepatic impairment.[2]

Approximately 75 percent of the immunoglobulins in the plasma are of the IgG fraction. This is the only immunoglobulin that crosses the placenta, providing maternal antibodies to the fetus and thus to neonates. IgG antibodies act against protein antigens, and account for most of the acquired antibodies active against bacteria, toxins, and viruses. IgG also activates the complement system.[8]

IgA constitutes approximately 20 percent of the immunoglobulin fraction, and is the prominent immunoglobulin in external secretions of the nasobronchial passages, gastrointestinal tract, and genitourinary system. Secretory IgA has antibody activity against bacterial and viral agents, toxins, and dietary macromolecules.[8]

IgM is prominent in the early immune response and includes antibodies against gram-negative bacteria, ABO isoagglutinins, autoantibodies, and cold agglutinins.[8]

IgD and IgE are present only in small amounts. IgD may play an important role in the binding of antigen to B lymphocytes. IgE has an important role in the immediate allergic or hypersensitivity reaction.[8]

The complement system consists of at least 15 plasma proteins. These proteins interact sequentially to mediate several functions of the inflammatory response, and work closely with antibodies in the body's immune system.[8]

BLOOD COAGULATION

With the exception of fibrinogen, only trace amounts of the clotting proteins are present in the blood. However, these trace proteins are responsible for transforming fibrinogen into a firm fibrin clot, and are essential for normal blood coagulation (hemostasis).

Figure 2-2 depicts the three steps in normal hemostasis. First, damaged blood vessels constrict to slow the flow of blood. Second, platelets are attracted to the area of damage, and aggregate to form a temporary platelet plug. The platelets forming this primary hemostatic plug disaggregate after 12 to 24 hours, and the plug does not re-form. Thus, platelets provide initial, but only temporary, control of bleeding from small vessels. Permanent hemostasis depends upon fibrin clot formation. This slot seals the damaged blood vessels until healing is complete.

The number of platelets in the blood stream usually ranges from 150,000 to 400,000/mm^3. When platelets are activated, they extend pseudopodia, which adhere to damaged subendothelial connective tissues and then aggregate, forming the platelet plug.[9] If a patient has either a decreased number of platelets (thrombocytopenia) or dysfunctional platelets, abnormal bleeding is possible.

A patient with fewer than 100,000 platelets/mm^3 has thrombocytopenia; this results from decreased platelet production (usually due to bone-marrow disease or to a vitamin B_{12} or folate deficiency), increased platelet destruction, or the dilution of platelets owing to massive transfusion. Depending upon the presence or absence of trauma and the effectiveness of existing platelets, patients with varying degrees of thrombocytopenia may have abnormal bleeding owing to the inability to form a platelet plug. Patients who have not had surgery or trauma, and who have well-functioning platelets, may experience a decrease in the platelet count to 5,000 platelets/mm^3 or less before abnormal bleeding occurs. Conversely, a patient with a normal platelet count may still be incapable of forming a platelet plug if the platelets do not aggregate properly.

The Ivy template bleeding time is the most reliable test of platelet function.[10] In this test, two carefully calibrated cuts are made on the forearm. The length of time necessary for the capilliaries to stop oozing blood is recorded as the bleeding time. From 2 to 8 minutes is considered normal. Bleeding times of 15 to 30 minutes or even longer may be found in patients with von Willebrand's disease and other diseases affecting platelet-function.

Since the platelet plug is temporary, normal clotting factors are also essential for hemostatis. There are 10 clotting proteins that interact sequentially to form a fibrin clot. Figure 2-3 shows the two possible pathways of clotting activation. One, called the extrinsic pathway, is apparently activated by a tissue factor released from damaged tissue. The intrinsic pathway is set into play when factor XII is activated by contact with collagen and elastin in the subendothelium of damaged blood vessels.[9]

If any of the clotting factors is missing or abnormal, there will be interference with normal clot formation. The normal activity range of most clotting factors is from 50 to 150 percent of their normal average activity. The relative

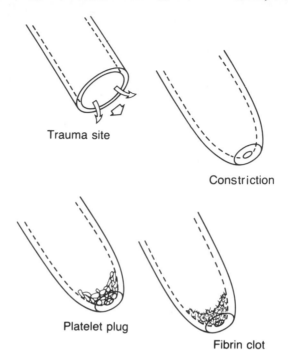

Trauma site

Constriction

Platelet plug

Fibrin clot

Fig. 2-2.   The sequence of events in normal hemostasis is: constriction of damaged blood vessels, platelet plug formation, and fibrin clot formation.

activity of a particular plasma sample is measured by comparing it with the activity of a pooled normal plasma sample, obtained by pooling the blood of 30 normal blood donors. Decreased levels of certain clotting factors may occur in liver disease, disseminated intravascular coagulation, and in patients having autoimmune antibodies. Congenital abnormalities of any of the clotting factors may also occur, and of these, hemophilia A (factor VIII deficiency) is the most common. The next most common abnormalities are hemophilia B (factor IX deficiency) and von Willebrand's disease (combined factor VIII deficiency and a platelet defect). The congenital clotting factor abnormalities are usually detected through a careful bleeding history and a family history. However, specific clotting factor assays are necessary for making the actual diagnosis.

Significant bleeding problems due to abnormal vasculature are extremely rare, but such collagen disorders as Ehlers-Danlos syndrome will occasionally result in defective blood vessels. Hereditary hemorrhagic telangiectasia and Henoch-Schönlein syndrome can also cause vessel wall abnormalities.[11] The friability of vessels can be noted at the time of surgery.

IMMUNOHEMATOLOGY

ABO System

Immunohematology addresses those aspects of hematology important to blood banking. The blood of every donor and recipient is classified as belonging

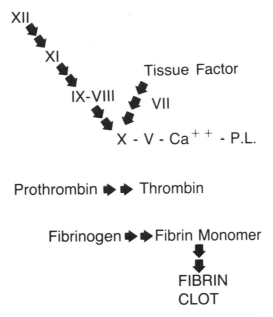

Fig. 2-3.   Simplified diagram of clotting pathway. There are 10 clotting proteins involved in a sequence of reactions which result in the formation of a fibrin clot.

to one of four types in the ABO system: A, B, AB, or O. In persons of Western European origin, about 46 percent have type O blood, 40 percent have type A, 10 percent have type B, and 4 percent have type AB.

The ABO blood type is based on the antigen found on an individual's erythrocytes and the antibodies found in the individual's serum. The ABO type of the individual is determined by testing his or her erythrocytes with two antisera: anti-A and anti-B. The blood type is confirmed by testing the individual's serum against known A and B red cells; nearly all individuals produce naturally occurring antibodies against A or B antigens not present on their own erythrocytes. Table 2-1 lists the antigens and antibodies for each blood type.

Whenever possible, patients are transfused with blood of their own ABO type. If necessary, type O blood can be given to patients of blood type A or B, but the donor plasma should be removed to prevent anti-A and anti-B antibodies from destroying the recipient's red cells. Type AB recipients can receive red cells from donors of blood type A or B. Anti-B antibodies in the blood of type A donors is rarely capable of destroying the recipient's red cells, but in cases of such transfusions it is still preferable to remove the plasma from the donor blood.[12]

Rh System

After the ABO system, the next most important genetic system for blood transfusion therapy is the Rh system. The most immunogenic antigen in this system is called D (or RH_0). If the patient has the D antigen, the patient's blood is

TABLE 2-1.   Routine ABO Blood Typing

Type	Red Cell Reactions with Antisera		Plasma (Serum) Reactions With Red Cells of A and B Types	
	Anti-A	Anti-B	A	B
O	−	−	+	+
A	+	−	−	+
B	−	+	+	−
AB	+	+	−	−

labeled Rh positive, and the patient can receive either Rh positive or Rh negative blood of the appropriate type. However, if the patient lacks the D antigen, the blood is Rh negative, and blood should be received only from Rh-negative donors. In contrast to the case in the ABO system, antibodies to the Rh antigens do not occur unless an Rh negative patient has been transfused previously with blood containing the specific antigen, or has delivered an Rh-positive child.

Other Blood Group Systems

There are 19 blood group systems in addition to the ABO and Rh systems. These 19 systems include approximately 300 antigens that can be detected on human red blood cells through the use of specific antibodies.[13] These antibodies make it unsafe to give blood that has been typed for ABO and Rh but has not been crossmatched, particularly to patients who have previously been transfused or have been pregnant.

Importance of the Crossmatch

The primary purpose of the blood crossmatch or compatibility test is to prevent transfusion reactions. Severe reactions result in hemolysis of transfused erythrocytes and may be life-threatening. There are also mild reactions that have no visible clinical signs but cause the rapid elimination of the donor's cells from the recipient's circulation. Thus, compatibility testing ensures that a patient benefits from a transfusion.[14]

A crossmatch normally includes an incubation phase and an antiglobulin (Coombs) test. These steps must be completed in order to detect all possible antibodies. An emergency crossmatch is very limited, and confirms only the ABO and Rh type. Since harmful antibodies may go undetected, an emergency crossmatch should not be ordered unless it is absolutely necessary.

PROCESSING OF BLOOD AND BLOOD COMPONENTS

Blood drawn into double or triple bags connected by sterile tubing can be separated into various components. If blood is drawn into a bag with two satellite bags attached, three different components can be obtained. If the blood is drawn into a bag with one satellite bag attached, the unit can be separated into two components.

With the triple bag system, platelets, cryoprecipitate (concentrated factor VIII and fibrinogen), and modified whole blood (blood that has had one or more components removed) can be obtained. With the double bag system, one can prepare platelets and modified whole blood, cryoprecipitate and modified whole blood, or packed red blood cells and fresh frozen plasma.

Medical staff often ask if any problems are caused by administering modified whole blood rather than whole blood to a patient. The removal of platelets and cryoprecipitate is actually a salvage process. The platelets in whole blood clump and lose their viability within 24 hours. The factor VIII level in refrigerated whole blood is significantly decreased at the end of 3 days, although in most cases this is not a problem for the recipient, because the factor VIII level is usually elevated in a patient under stress from surgery or injury. Most patients also have sufficient platelet reserves, exceptions being the patient who has had a massive transfusion (more than about 15 units of blood in a 24 hour period), or the patient who has a disease process involving the platelets. In such cases, thrombocytopenia may cause bleeding. In patients with diffuse microvascular bleeding, dilutional thrombocytopenia is the most common cause of abnormal bleeding.[15]

Although experimentation is being done on oxygen-carrying compounds that might be used as blood substitutes, human donors are at present the only source of blood and blood products. In order to make safe and effective use of the blood and blood components available, medical staff must know: (a) the functions of blood and its constituents; (b) the conditions that compromise function of the various components (such as disease states, storage time and so forth); (c) the indications for use of blood and specific blood components; and (d) the possible complications of blood component therapy.

REFERENCES

1. Lewis SM: The constituents of normal blood. In: Blood and Its Disorders, ed. Hardisty, RM and Wetherall, DJ. London, Blackwell Scientific Publications, 1974. p 3
2. Dougherty WM: Introduction to Hematology, 2d edn. St. Louis, C.V. Mosby, 1976. pp 53, 54, 124–125, 126, 114
3. Beutler E: Erythrocyte metabolism and maintenance of erythrocytes. In: Hematology, 2d edn. Williams WJ et al. New York, McGraw-Hill, 1977. pp 126, 178–183
4. Bryan-Brown CW, Valeri CR, Altschule MD: The coloring substance of blood. Crit Care Med, 7(9):358, 1979
5. Perutz MF: Hemoglobin structure and respiratory transport. Scientific American, 239(6):95, 96, 103–105, 106, 1978
6. Dale DC: Abnormalities of leukocytes. In: Harrison's Principles of Internal Medicine, ed. Isselbacher, KJ et al. New York, McGraw-Hill, 1980. p 284, 290
7. Applebaum F et al.: White Cell Syllabus. University of Washington, 1979. pp 16–18, 33–38, 51–52

8. Gilliand BC: Introduction to clinical immunology. In: Harrison's Principles of Internal Medicine, ed. Isselbacher, KJ et al. New York, McGraw-Hill, 1980. pp 316, 318, 322

9. Thompson AR et al.: Hemostasis and Thrombosis Syllabus. University of Washington, 1980. pp 8–12

10. Mielke CH et al.: The standardized normal Ivy bleeding time. Blood, 34:204–215, 1969

11. Nossel HL: Bleeding disorders due to vessel wall abnormalities. In: Harrison's Principles of Internal Medicine, ed. Isselbacher, KJ et al. New York, McGraw-Hill, 1980. pp 1559–1560

12. Giblett ER: Erythrocyte antigens and antibodies. In: Hematology, 2d edn., ed. Williams, WJ et al. New York, McGraw-Hill, 1977. p 1498

13. Giblett, ER: Blood groups and blood transfusion. In: Harrison's Principles of Internal Medicine, ed. Isselbacher, KJ et al. New York, McGraw-Hill, 1980. p 1568

14. Levine P: Blood Group Antigens and Antibodies as Applied to Compatibility Testing. New Jersey, Ortho Diagnostics, 1967. p 3

15. Counts RB et al.: Hemostasis in massively transfused trauma patients. Ann Surg, 190(1):91, 1979

3 | Hemodynamic Monitoring as an Assessment and Management Tool

Mary Farley

The incidence of extensive surgical procedures on older and high risk patients, as well as the operative survival and rapid mobilization of traumatized patients, has increased. Favorable patient outcome has been enhanced by the parallel use of sophisticated hemodynamic monitoring procedures.

Hemodynamic monitoring is the observation of the response of the cardiovascular system to illness, injury, and treatment. In this chapter, indications for the use of both invasive and noninvasive monitoring techniques will be described. The observations used to assess the cardiovascular status of the patient at four locations—prehospital, in the emergency room, in the operative suite, and in the intensive care ward—will be discussed. The location of the patient determines the therapy used for patient revival, and these efforts will be referred to as levels of resuscitation. The limitations, the complications, and the use of the information derived from hemodynamic measurement, as well as nursing responsibilities attendant upon such monitoring, will also be considered.

The purpose of hemodynamic monitoring is to assess the degree of compromise of the circulation in the critically ill, and to guide ongoing therapy. Monitoring provides information about vascular capacity, blood volume, pump efficiency, and tissue perfusion.[1] The level of sophistication of monitoring is determined by the logistics of location, personnel, and available equipment, and by the indications for escalating the invasiveness of the monitoring devices used.

At each stage in the assessment and management of the critically ill, the following questions must be answered: (a) What parameter must be measured? (b) Why do we need to have this information? (c) When do we need to have it? (d) How are we going to measure the required parameter? (e) Where is the best anatomical place to measure it?

Monitoring of the patient with cardiovascular and intravascular volume compromise may be considered in terms of a pyramid of increasing complexity and procedural invasiveness. The base of the pyramid constitutes the foundation upon which the other levels are built (Fig. 3-1).

The passage of time is required in order to detect alterations in cardiovascular dynamics in the physical examination. Thus, since common clinical findings are "slow" indicators of biologic change,[2,3] clinical signs of hypovolemia and circulatory compromise are of limited value in this regard.

Escalation of the extent and invasiveness of monitoring is indicated in states of continued hypoperfusion; such monitoring includes the placing of urinary catheters, the taking of electrocardiograms, the monitoring of central venous pressure (CVP), and the analysis of blood and urine. The hemodynamic monitoring of renal blood flow comprises measurement of the minute or hourly urine volume, demonstrating the kidney's ability to concentrate wastes.[4] The CVP can be a reliable approximation of the efficacy of the right ventricle in handling venous return, and is an index of blood volume if myocardial function and vascular tone are normal. Since the CVP is a measure of dynamic relationships between these parameters, the volume status cannot be determined from a single CVP reading; serial measurements of the CVP response to fluid boluses are more valuable.[5] Electrocardiograms give information on heart rate and rhythm from which inferences about stroke volume and cardiac output can be made. Blood and urine specimens are used as hemodynamic measurements to indicate volume loss and to guide fluid replacement.

During subsequent surgery, there may be continued massive hemorrhage, fluid shifts, acid–base derangements, and prolonged periods under anesthesia, requiring the taking of multiple blood samples and the intensive monitoring of volume status and cardiorespiratory performance for effective hemodynamic monitoring. Arterial line and pulmonary artery catheters are used to augment CVPs and urine volume during surgery. Patients with pre-existing cardiopulmonary disease, as well as those with traumatic injuries requiring massive fluid replacement, are candidates for this sophisticated intraoperative hemodynamic monitoring.

Admission to surgical intensive care units for continued, extensive monitoring is indicated for those patients who (a) have severe multisystem injury; (b) have required multiple transfusions of stored blood; (c) have signficant preexisting cardiovascular, pulmonary, or renal disease; (d) have marked sepsis; (e) have a strong possibility of pulmonary or cardiac injury; and (f) have had prolonged periods of hypotension. The goals of therapy are to replenish extracellular fluid without overloading the patient, to preserve organ function, and to prevent further organ injury from the patient's disease or secondary to treatment.[5]

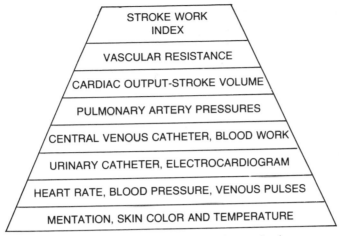

Fig. 3-1. Levels of hemodynamic monitoring

In critically ill surgical patients, recognition of the extent of fluid loss and estimation of the fluid volume required for resuscitation is difficult. Such patients have tube drainage, wound drainage, diarrheal and third-space losses, and the internal pooling of blood in hematomas. Third-space losses[7,8] derive from prolonged hypovolemia leading to altered cell membrane function and a subsequent shift of intracellular and extracellular electrolytes resulting in cellular swelling. Shires and co-workers have demonstrated a loss of "functional extracellular volume" in prolonged hemorrhagic shock.[6] These fluid shifts result in secondary loss of intravascular volume, and potentiate the primary volume deficit.

An evaluation of the amount of fluid available for circulation, as well as of the ability of the cardiovascular system to circulate this fluid adequately, includes an assessment of the efficiency of the heart. Cardiac performance may be decreased by lack of blood volume or by myocardial insufficiency, either as a direct result of inadequate perfusion for a prolonged period or secondary to the use of anesthetic agents.[9] As many as 2 percent of patients without previous evidence of coronary artery disease develop myocardial infarction during or immediately after a major surgical procedure.[10] Thus, preservation of adequate cardiac function is one of the most important factors in the outcome of critically ill patients. Inadequate cardiac function for even a relatively short period results in deterioration of the function of other organ systems. The use of cardiac filling pressures has been recommended in the evaluation of cardiovascular dynamics in critically ill patients.[11-13] Centrally located catheters enhance the ability of the physician and nurse to prevent complications, and to continually diagnose, assess, and therapeutically manage hemodynamic problems.[14]

Central Venous Pressure Monitoring

The central venous pressure reflects right ventricular end-diastolic pressure, or right ventricular filling pressure (preload). Preload indicates the venous filling pressure, and it is measured clinically via a CVP line or pulmonary artery catheter; the preload pressure is determined by blood volume and venous capacitance or tone, and from the pumping action of the heart.[15]

The CVP can be increased or decreased by the circulating blood volume, by vasoconstriction, or by decreased myocardial contractility.[16] The CVP can rise when venous return and venous tone increase, or when cardiac function deteriorates; under the opposite circumstances, the CVP decreases. However, CVP levels are often misleading; an elevated CVP may be found in hypovolemia, while the patient continues to be fluid depleted, if the patient is on positive pressure ventilation or has preexisting or traumatic pulmonary disease. Indeed, patients may be grossly overloaded with fluid, especially crystalloid, to the point of pulmonary edema, and a normal CVP reading may still be obtained.[4,17-19] The inaccuracy of the CVP is frequently found in disease states characterized by changes in pulmonary vascular resistance (PVR), such as chronic obstructive pulmonary disease (COPD) or cor pulmonale, as well as diseases associated with cardiac valve destruction or impaired left ventricular function, such as myocardial ischemia or infarction.[20]

Serial CVP measurements in response to boluses of intravenous fluids are valuable in the patient with nondisparate ventricular function. A depressed or normal CVP that does not rise significantly with rapid administration of a balanced salt solution is usually indicative of a continuing hypovolemia. The diagnosis can be supported by the demonstration of a measured decrease in cardiac output with administration of the solution.[9]

CVP measurements are indicated when information is needed about right ventricular performance and venous return. The right atrial mean pressure ($\overline{RAP}$) is needed to calculate the systemic vascular resistance (SVR), which is an estimate of afterload. Afterload basically reflects the resistance to left ventricular emptying that is referred to as impedance. Afterload is measured clinically from blood pressure and systemic vascular resistance (SVR) recordings, and requires the use of a pulmonary artery catheter[15] (Fig. 3-2).

In those patients with hypovolemia, normal cardiac function, and relatively normal pulmonary function, the CVP remains an acceptable guide to blood volume. The catheter for CVP monitoring must be positioned properly, as verified by x-ray, and measurement techniques must be accurate. A zero reference level must be established and used for all subsequent measurements. The phlebostatic axis, as illustrated in an article by Woods, is recommended.[21] The measurement instrument used, either water- or mercury-based, should be free of air and blood clots, and the column of fluid should fall freely and fluctuate with respiration. Blood drawing from the CVP catheter should be avoided in order to decrease the risk of infection, and all stopcocks should be tightly secured to decrease the chances of air embolization and hemorrhage. Other complications of CVP lines include arrhythmias, perforation of the atrium or right ventricle during catheter insertion, thrombophlebitis, thrombosis with a blood clot or with the catheter tip, and pneumothorax if insertion of the catheter is via a subclavian or jugular vein.[4,22] Unilateral pulmonary edema and cerebral hyperosmolar insult have been reported from CVP infusions through catheters introduced into the

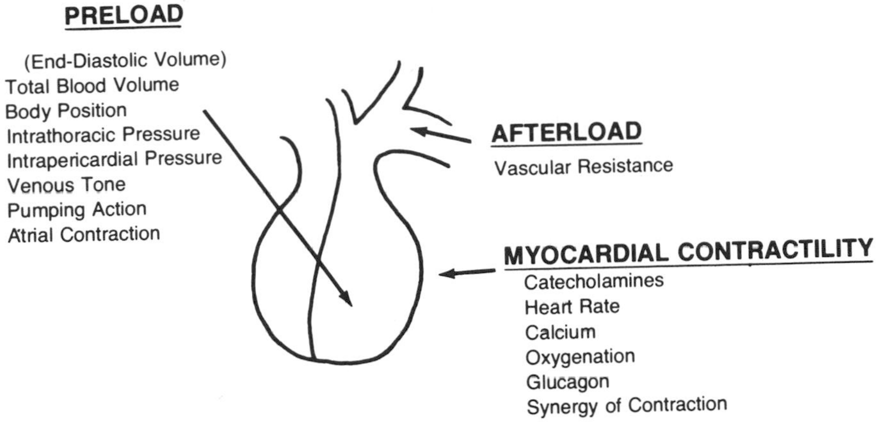

PRELOAD

(End-Diastolic Volume)
Total Blood Volume
Body Position
Intrathoracic Pressure
Intrapericardial Pressure
Venous Tone
Pumping Action
Atrial Contraction

AFTERLOAD

Vascular Resistance

MYOCARDIAL CONTRACTILITY

Catecholamines
Heart Rate
Calcium
Oxygenation
Glucagon
Synergy of Contraction

Fig. 3-2. Parameters of myocardial function

internal jugular system.[23] The most frequent complication of CVP measurement is improper fluid therapy based on incorrect measurement due to the use of an incorrect zero reference point, or to air or clots in the catheter resulting in a damped waveform.[1]

Patients with severe, acute cardiopulmonary decompensation, massive trauma, or concomitant septic shock require more extensive monitoring. In these patients, a pulmonary artery thermodilution catheter is indicated.[9,24,25]

Pulmonary Artery Pressure Monitoring

Pulmonary artery monitoring facilitates the treatment of patients who require large-volume fluid replacements or drug therapy to maximize cardiac function. The use of pulmonary artery catheters is aimed at achieving adequate circulatory volume and adequate perfusion pressures without cardiac decompensation and resultant pulmonary edema.

The pulmonary artery catheter is inserted through a cutdown, or percutaneously into the antecubital vein or, more commonly, through the subclavian or jugular veins (see refs. 1, 26–28). Passage of the catheter within the right heart and into the pulmonary artery is directed by the drag of blood on the inflated balloon at the catheter tip. The position of the catheter in the vena cava, right atrium, right ventricle, and pulmonary artery is monitored by observing the changes in pressure waveforms on the oscilloscope at the patient's bedside. The nursing responsibilities for pulmonary artery catheter insertion include preparation of the patient by adequate explanation, careful checking for electrical hazards, assurance of balloon integrity, equipment assembly, and prewarming of transducers and oscilloscopes.

The design of the pulmonary artery thermodilution catheter permits the measurement of raw hemodynamic data and the calculation of indices that affect cardiac performance and tissue perfusion (Table 3-2). The catheter has a quadruple-lumen design: lumen one is the distal lumen, which terminates at the

TABLE 3-1.   List of Abbreviations for Hemodynamic Values

$\overline{BP}$	Mean Arterial Blood Pressure
CI	Cardiac Index
CO	Cardiac Output
CVP	Central Venous Pressure
HR	Heart Rate
LA	Left Atrial
LVEDP	Left Ventricular End-Diastolic Pressure
PA	Pulmonary Artery
PAP	Pulmonary Artery Pressure
PAEDP	Pulmonary Artery End-Diastolic Pressure
PAWP	Pulmonary Artery Wedge Pressure
PVR	Pulmonary Vascular Resistance
$\overline{RAP}$	Right Atrial Mean Pressure
SV	Stroke Volume
SVR	Systemic Vascular Resistance
SWI	Stroke Work Index

tip of the catheter and allows measurement of chamber pressures; pulmonary artery (PAP), and pulmonary artery wedge pressure (PAWP), as well as providing access for mixed venous sampling for the calculation of pulmonary shunt fractions; lumen two is the proximal lumen, which terminates 25 to 30 centimeters from the catheter tip, and is located in the right atrium when the distal lumen is in the pulmonary artery. The proximal lumen allows measurement of the right atrial mean pressure ($\overline{RAP}$), which is the equivalent of the CVP, but which is measured in millimeters of mercury (mmHg = torr) rather than in centimeters of water (cm H_2O). A single transducer can be used to monitor both $\overline{RA}$ and PA pressures. The proximal lumen is also the entry port for the injectate used to measure cardiac output (CO). Lumen three is the balloon lumen, which serves for inflation and deflation of the balloon at the distal end of the catheter. The fourth lumen contains the electrical wires and the thermistor bead, which is positioned on the catheter surface approximately 4 centimeters from the catheter tip.[29]

Lumens one and two of the thermodilution catheter must be continuously flushed with a heparinized solution—either dextrose and water or saline—in order to assure their patency. The port terminal of the distal lumen of the catheter is connected to a heparinized solution.

In our surgical intensive care unit, a Sorenson Special Pressure Monitoring line is connected to a Sorenson C.F.S. Intraflow continuous flush device, which irrigates the catheter with 3 or 4 cc of solution per minute, and allows intermittent flushing of the catheter. Two stopcocks are connected to the Intraflow device and connected to the catheter: one for clearing the line prior to blood-drawing, the other for drawing blood specimens. A male-to-male, 6-inch, Medex pressure monitoring line is used to connect the proximal lumen of the catheter to the monitoring system. Another stopcock is inserted into the proximal lumen for blood drawing and for cardiac output determinations, and the entire system is then connected to the transducer (see Fig. 3-3).

With the use of high pressure tubing, the transducer of the pulmonary artery catheter may be mounted with a movable arm (which incorporates a carpenter's level for accuracy of the phlebostatic level determination) on an intravenous

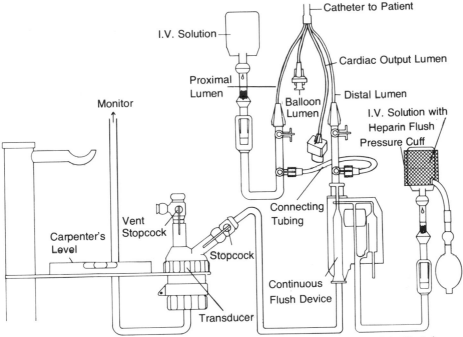

Fig. 3-3. Standard pulmonary artery monitoring setup; designed by Eric H. Johnson, R.N., Harborview Medical Center, Seattle, Washington

pole. Alternatively, the transducer can be directly connected to stopcocks and mounted on an armboard. The armboard can be padded with towels to build the height of the transducer to the phlebostatic level, and can be left at the patient's side. After calibration of the pressure module, and with the transducer correctly leveled, hemodynamic pressures can be measured and new physiologic data becomes available for therapy of the patient.

In the absence of pulmonary stenosis, the PA systolic pressure is equal to the right ventricular pressure during systole.[30] The PA pressure increases with increased PVR or increased pulmonary flow, and is frequently elevated in COPD patients.[31] The PA end-diastolic pressure (PAEDP) is approximately the same as the PAWP when the PVR is normal and when the patient is not mechanically ventilated or is not on high levels of positive end-expiratory pressure (PEEP).[16] A PEEP of greater than or equal to 10 cm H_2O may cause a preload-reducing effect in some patients.[32-36] In the absence of mitral valve disease, the PAWP approximates the left atrial (LA) and left ventricular end-diasytolic pressures (LVEDP).

When the balloon of the pulmonary artery catheter is inflated, a column of fluid exists from the pulmonary capillary to the left atrium, and the pressure in the left ventricle at end-diastole should therefore be approximately equal to the pressure in the pulmonary capillaries. In patients with normal left ventricular compliance, an increase in the LVEDP indicates an increase in left ventricular volume; a decrease in the LVEDP indicates a decrease in left ventricular volume. Changes in the PAWP give early indications of left ventricular function, and they are used to guide therapy.[37] Changes in the PAWP may precede by hours x-ray or ausculatory findings suggestive of left ventricular decompensation.[38]

The PAWP alone is an inadequate criterion for severely ill patients; the addition of cardiac output monitoring allows more adequate measurement of the hemodynamic status of these patients.[39,40]

Cardiac Output

The cardiac output, expressed in liters per minute, is the volume of blood pumped by the heart. With knowledge of the volume of cold fluid injected, the temperature difference between the fluid and the blood, and the thermistor calibration factor, the cardiac output can be determined electronically by a bedside computer. The output must be interpreted in reference to the size of the individual by calculating the cardiac index (CI) with a Dubois body-surface-area chart. The cardiac output must also be interpreted in relation to the patient's disease process. Sepsis may cause hyperdynamic states with cardiac outputs as much as double the normal range.[39,41]

The accuracy of cardiac output measurement depends on careful technique in measuring the amount of injectate, in the rapidity of the injection—which should not take longer than 10 seconds from the time the syringe is removed from the cooling solution to the completion of the injection (when using iced solutions)—and in the timing of each injection so that it occurs during the same phase of the respiratory cycle, preferably during expiration. Edwards Laboratories recommends taking three measurements and using a computed mean value of these. If properly performed, the measurements should not vary more than 10 percent.[4,42] During cardiac output measurement, any intravenous lines should be moved to sites other than that being used for the pulmonary artery catheter so as to avoid bolus effects from infused medications.

Use of the Information

The PAWP and cardiac output can be used to construct Starling curves; alternatively, indices calculated from these measurements can be used to construct ventricular function curves (Fig. 3-4). The Frank-Starling law states that the muscle of the heart can stretch and contract with greater force (up to a limit) when an increased volume of blood is brought to the heart from the peripheral circulation. An increase in the PAWP results in an increase in cardiac output within the physiologic limits of the myocardium. The optimal filling pressure for seriously ill patients is believed to be that at which the cardiac output is maximal. The exception to this occurs with those patients who have acute respiratory insufficiency from "leaky pulmonary capillaries." For these patients, the filling pressure may have to be reduced in order to maximize oxygenation.[39]

In uncomplicated hypovolemia there will be decreases in the following measurements: the CI, $\overline{RAP}$, and PAWP, and usually also in the systemic arterial pressure. Volume replacement can be guided by changes in the PAWP and

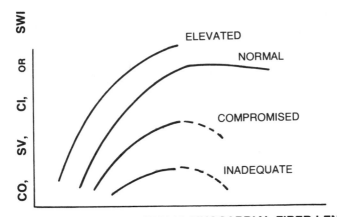

PAWP, LVEDP, OR DIASTOLIC MYOCARDIAL FIBER LENGTH

Fig. 3-4. Ventricular function curves

cardiac output. Return of the PAWP to the normal range of from 6 to 12 torr is usually sufficient. Elevation of the PAWP to from 15 to 18 torr results in an increased cardiac output in most patients. However, pulmonary artery wedge pressures of greater than 18 torr may cause pulmonary congestion with no change in cardiac output.[43]

The return of the cardiac output and PAWP to normal values may be difficult to achieve in critically ill patients. When the indices of ventricular function—stroke volume (SV), cardiac index (CI), systemic vascular resistance (SVR), pulmonary vascular resistance (PVR), and stroke work index (SWI)—are known, these parameters can be manipulated to improve tissue perfusion. The indices of these parameters also give additional information on preload, myocardial contractility, and afterload.

The stroke volume is determined by many factors, including filling pressures, ventricular distensibility, mean arterial pressure ($\overline{BP}$), or SVR, and myocardial contractility. Changes in any of these factors may affect the cardiac output. Both the SVR and the PVR are measures of vessel impedance to blood flow, and are affected by catecholamines, extrinsic pressures surrounding the vessels, and intrinsic volume. The stroke work index is a measure of how hard the heart muscle must work to pump the blood. The SWI is affected by the volume status, SVR, oxygenation, and heart rate of the patient.

Calculation of the foregoing indices and serial evaluation of ventricular performance curves, helps in the assessment of not only the initial hemodynamic status of the patient but also his response to therapeutic intervention or to spontaneous changes in cardiovascular status.[44] Just as the cardiac output differs among patients, so do performance curves vary. Therefore, it is necessary to obtain these curves for each patient in order to determine his "optimal filling pressure," and to then maintain that level by adjustment of fluid or drug therapy.[39] However, all such measurements must be interpreted in light of the clinical situation.

A flow or recording sheet must be designed that will deal with the hemodynamic monitoring data that are generated. The sheet must allow sequential review of the information and a trend analysis of the monitored indices; the sheet should include the date, time, and indices measured, as well as columns for IV fluid rates, vasoactive drug drip rates, levels of PEEP, urine output, and an additional column for comments regarding fluid boluses, PEEP trials, and other patient-care manipulations. The flow sheet must include formulas for calculating the indices derived from the various measurements, and it is helpful if the sheet includes normal values. It is imperative that the same cardiac index calculated from the Dubois chart be used in all subsequent calculations if hemodynamic trends are to be interpreted in terms of therapy, and not in terms of weight gain from fluid administration (for a copy of our institutions flow sheet, please contact the author). Table 3-2 provides normal values and formulas for calculating the various hemodynamic indices.

The nursing management of patients with pulmonary artery lines in place includes prevention of infection through daily dressing changes and 48-hour IV fluid and tubing changes.[45,46] Continuous monitoring of waveforms with lines that are air and clot free, thorough flushing and capping of all stopcocks after blood drawing, and careful attention to use of the same zero reference point are all mandatory for safe and accurate monitoring. The transducer used for monitoring should be balanced, and the pressure module calibrated frequently (at least once per shift), flushed daily with IV solution, kept blood and air free, and changed during septic episodes.[47] Air must be put carefully into the balloon lumen to avoid damage to the intima of the pulmonary vessel and to avoid balloon rupture. Potentially lethal complications of pulmonary artery catheterization are possible, but can be avoided by conscientious attention to details; Table 3-3 lists the potential complications of such catheterization.

Arterial Pressure Monitoring

Arterial pressure monitoring is useful in unstable patients, since, particularly in the hypotensive patient, it is frequently impossible to obtain accurate arterial cuff pressure measurements or reliable arterial blood. Cuff methods are unreliable because the diminished pulsatile flow in low flow states may fail to produce a sound wave, and Korotkoff's sounds are thus lost. Disappearance of peripheral pulses is probably the result of a reduced stroke volume and of an altered arterial-wall stiffness. Nevertheless, patients with all of the peripheral manifestations of shock may have normal intraarterial pressure despite reduced cuff pressures. Thus, failure to recognize that a low cuff pressure does not necessarily indicate arterial hypotension may lead to errors in therapy.[48]

Intraarterial monitoring, with the transducer mounted at the level of the left atrium, provides an accurate reflection of systolic, diastolic, and mean pressure. It also permits the continuous monitoring of beat-to-beat changes in pressure. Since the coronary artery pressure depends primarily upon the diastolic blood pressure, it is desirable, for hypotensive patients,[49] to provide a method for accurate recording of the mean arterial and diastolic pressures. The mean arterial pressure measurement is necessary for calculating the SVR and SWI. Arterial cannulation is also less disturbing to the patient, and allows repeated arterial

TABLE 3-2. Normal Hemodynamic Values and Formulas to Calculate Cardiac Output Indices

Normal Values		Formulas
Right arterial pressure	2–6 torr	measured
Right ventricular (systolic/diastolic)	20/5 torr	measured
Pulmonary artery wedge	5–12 torr mean	measured
Left atrial pressure	5–12 torr mean	inferred
Left ventricular end-diastolic pressure	5–12 torr, mean	inferred
Cardiac output	4–8 L/min	measured
Cardiac index	2.5–3.5 L/min/m²	$CI = CO \div BSA$
Stroke volume	60–70 ml/beat	$SV = CO \div HR \times 1000$
Stroke work index	50–70 gm/min/m²	$SWI = (\overline{BP} - \overline{PAWP}) \div \dfrac{CI \times 13.6}{HR}$
Systemic vascular resistance	900–1200 dynes/sec/cm⁻⁵	$SVR = \overline{BP} - \overline{RAP} \times 80 \div CO$
Pulmonary vascular resistance	150–250 dynes/sec/cm⁻⁵	$PVR = \overline{PAP} - \overline{PAWP} \times 80 \div CO$

Forrester JS, Diamond G, Chatterjee K: Medical therapy of acute myocardial infarction by application of hemodynamic subsets. N Engl J Med, 295:1404–1413, 1976. Bland R, Shoemaker WC, Shabbot MM: Physiologic monitoring goals for the critically ill patient. Surg, Gynecol Obstet, 147:833–841, 1978. Reprinted, by permission of The New England Journal of Medicine (295:1404–1413, 1976).

sampling of blood gases in a steady state, thus avoiding acute changes in blood-gas tension that may confuse the interpretation of results obtained from intermittent puncture.[5] Arterial cannulation also avoids the error of venous admixture in gas sampling, which can occur with an arteriovenous fistula and which may markedly lower arterial oxygen values.[50] Arterial cannulation is indicated for patients who require four or more blood gas samplings per day.

The pulse configuration given by a properly functioning catheter, with a properly calibrated transducer and oscilloscope, can provide a rough estimate of left ventricular function. A rapid upstroke and full contour usually represent an effectively contracting ventricle and adequate volume; the pressure curve of a failing ventricle may have a low amplitude and slower upstroke configuration. Cardiac arrhythmias alter the filling time, and therefore decrease the end-diastolic volume and stroke volume, with this decrease being reflected in the arterial pressure tracing. The arterial pressure line thus allows continuous evaluation of blood pressure, and gives information related to ventricular function for observation of drug effect and volume manipulation.[9,51]

The equipment assembly for arterial pressure monitoring includes a pressurized-heparinized line identical to that used for the PA catheter, with the substitution of one stopcock, and an Abbot 5-inch extension set with a "T" connector onto the Sorenson Intraflow; the T connector is connected directly to the arterial cannula (see also ref. 52 for the line assembly.) The use of the T connector allows blood sampling through the rubber portal, and decreases displacement and contamination of the arterial cannula from the opening and

TABLE 3-3.   Potential Complications of
Pulmonary Artery Catheters

Pulmonary infarction
Rupture of a branch of the pulmonary artery
Atrial, ventricular arrhythmias
Balloon rupture
Intracardiac catheter knotting
Superior vena cava, intracardiac thrombus
Septal endocardial, valvular vegetations
Air embolism
Electrocution
Bundle branch block and complete heart block
Pulmonary valve injury

Adapted from: Baker, et al.: Surg Clin North Am
57:1139–1158, 1977. Thompson, et al.: Anesthesiology 51:359–362, 1979. O'Toole, et al.: N Engl J Med
301:1167–1168, 1979. Deren et al.: Thorax 34:550–
553, 1979.

closing of stopcocks. The prime location for contamination of the line is at the site of blood sampling.[53]

Cannulation is usually done in the radial or dorsalis pedis artery owing to the collateral circulation at these sites. When the radial artery is used, an Allen's test or Doppler evaluation of the palmar circulation must be done before introduction of the catheter in order to assure a patent ulnar artery.[54] Doppler measurement of the dorsalis pedis and posterior tibial circulation, or great toe blush, are required to assure adequate circulation to the foot.[55] These precautions are necessary in order to avoid serious compromise, from arterial catheterization, to the patient's circulation.

The three complications of greatest concern in arterial cannulation are clotting, exsanguination, and infection. Clotting can be prevented by continuous flushing of the catheter with the Sorenson Intraflow; the nurse must also check the circulation and pulse of the extremity every hour to assure adequacy of circulation. The monitor alarms should be set with high and low alarms, and must be turned on, since exsanguination is a real threat; blood loss through discon-nected 20-gauge catheters may be as much as 200 milliliters in a matter of 4 or 5 minutes.[26] Such loss can be prevented by the use of Luer-Lock connections, and by frequent checking of the sytem to ensure its intactness. The risk of sepsis may be decreased by changing the dressing and applying antibiotic ointment to the cannulation site daily. The dressing should be kept dry, and tubing and IV solutions should be changed at least every 48 hours.[45,56]

Thrombus formation occurs in from 20 to 40 percent of patients in whom a radial artery catheter is left in place for more than 12 to 18 hours.[4,57] The incidence of thrombosis is higher if the patient is critically ill, is hypercoagulable, or has impaired tissue perfusion from shock. Even without total occlusion of the radial artery, patients may develop digital gangrene in one or two digits secon-dary to embolization by fragments of intima, plaque, or of clot that forms on the catheter. Such emboli obstruct digital vessels peripheral to the catheter and cause the tissue loss that may result in gangrene. Skin necrosis proximal to the site of radial artery cannulation has been reported, and may be due to large-bore catheter use or to excessive flushing of the catheter line, which results in arterial spasm and reversal of flow in the artery.[58,59] During monitoring, the wrist should be extended or hyperextended and affixed to an armboard to ensure continuous stability of the catheter, and constant solution flow. Intermittent and manual flush systems should be avoided, since they increase the likelihood of thrombus formation from a clot of air; arterial emboli can be lethal if they travel centrally and reach the cerebral circulation.[26,60,61]

The incidence of thrombus formation increases with catheter size, as more of the arterial lumen becomes occluded. Less vascular occlusion has been found with the use of 20-gauge teflon catheters and constant irrigation with heparinized solutions.[62,63] The length of time during which the artery is cannulated is also a factor in arterial occlusion and catheter dysfunction, as demonstrated by inaccurate pulse pressures, poor tracings, and difficulty in drawing blood.[61] Nevertheless, with proper maintenance and care in the gathering of accurate data, arterial lines add much valuable information to the treatment of the critically ill patient.

Conclusion

Invasive hemodynamic monitoring procedures can add valuable information to patient care. With judicious use of these procedures, intelligent therapy can be instituted to ensure a successful outcome in as many patients as possible. In using these procedures, however, one must consider that they are not innocuous. They must be regarded as constituting a calculated risk, since a small but finite proportion of patients who are monitored by invasive techniques suffer untoward and occasionally catastrophic consequences.[4] Thus, the level of invasiveness of monitoring should be commensurate with the severity of the physiologic derangement, and the benefits of such monitoring should markedly outweigh the attendant risks of the technique.[51] Since significant risks and costs are incurred in gathering hemodynamic data, it must be accurate. The direct costs of the insertion of a pulmonary artery catheter alone, including the cost of the catheter, disposable supplies, and physicians fees, are in the range of $400 to $500 per insertion.[25]

Because of a tendency to observe the equipment, and not the patient, a danger in sophisticated hemodynamic monitoring is separation of the patient from the personnel responsible for his or her care. "Monitoring is intended to augment, not replace, bedside observation of critically ill patients by skilled physicians, nurses, and therapists."[5] It is useful to remember that the ultimate hemodynamic criterion in the treatment of the critically ill is the response of the patient, and not the monitoring data. The key to success rests with the team caring for the patient more than the equipment. Nevertheless, monitoring of all major systems is necessary for optimal care, and all levels of hemodynamic monitoring are important. In the words of Holliday, "The intensive care nurse is the indispensable component of the team; she must be knowledgeable, motivated, and enthusiastic, and must remain 'the complete monitor.'"[6]

REFERENCES

1. Woods SL, Grose BL: Hemodynamic monitoring in patients with acute myocardial infarction. In: Cardiovascular Nursing, eds. Underhill SL et al. Philadelphia, Lippincott. (In press)
2. Holder DA: Hemodynamic monitoring of the acutely ill patient. Can Med Assoc J, 121:895–935, 1979
3. Swan HJC, Ganz, W: Hemodynamic monitoring: a personal and historical perspective. Can Med Assoc J, 127:868–871, 1979
4. Baker RJ: Monitoring in critically ill patients. Surg Clin North Am, 57:1939–1158, 1977
5. Carrico CJ, Horowitz JH: Monitoring the critically ill surgical patient. In: Advances in Surgery. Chicago, Year Book Publishers, 1977
6. Holliday RL, Doris PJ: Monitoring the critically ill surgical patient. Can Med Assoc J, 127:931–935, 1979
7. Trunkey D, Holcroft J, Carpenter MA: Calcium flux during hemorrhagic shock in baboons. J Trauma, 16:633, 1979
8. Haljamäe H: Effects of hemorrhagic shock and treatment with hypothermia in the potassium content and transport of single mammalian skeletal muscle cells. Acta Physiol Scand, 78:189, 1970
9. Shires GT: Principles and management of hemorrhagic shock. In: Care of the Trauma Patient, ed. Shires GT. New York, McGraw-Hill, 1979
10. Dawber TR, Thomas HE: Prevention of myocardial infarction. Prog Cardiovasc Dis, 13:343, 1971
11. Cerra F, Milch R, Lajos R.: Pulmonary artery catheterization in critically ill surgical patients. Ann Surg, 177:37–39, 1973
12. Swan HJC, Ganz W: Use of balloon flotation catheters in critically ill patients. Surg Clin North Am, 55:501–520, 1975
13. Gilbertson AA: Pulmonary artery catheterization and wedge pressure measurements in the general intensive therapy unit. Br J Anaesth, 46:97–104, 1974
14. Hathaway RG: Description of Swan-Ganz catheter clinical indications, contraindications, precautions, complications. Nurs Clin North Am, 13:389–407, 1978
15. Haas JM: Understanding hemodynamic monitoring: concepts of preload and afterload. Critical Care Quarterly, 2:1–8, 1979
16. Forrester JS, Diamond G, Chatterjee K, et al.: Medical therapy of acute myocardial infarction by application of hemodynamic subsets. N Engl J Med, 295:1356–1362, 1976
17. DeMuth WE: CVP measurement in the injured patient. Penn Med, 79:55–59, 1976
18. Kay G, Kearns P: Monitoring central venous pressure: principles, procedures and problems. Can Nurse, 72:15–18, 1976
19. Tinker J: Two methods of assessing the critically ill patient. Nursing Times, 297:318–328, 1978
20. Bollish SJ, Foster TS: Swan-Ganz catheter: an important tool for monitoring drug therapy in the critically ill. Hospital Formulary, 15:99–116, 1980
21. Wood SL: Monitoring pulmonary artery pressures. Am J Nurs, 76:1765–1771, 1976
22. Adair R, Moyes M: Fatal complications of central venous catheters. Br Med J, 3:746–747, 1971
23. Royal HD, Shields JB, Donati RM: Misplacement of central venous pressure catheters and unilateral pulmonary edema. Arch Intern Med, 135:1502–1505, 1975

24. Tinker J: Two methods of assessing the critically ill patient. Nursing Times, 297:318–320, 1978
25. Dalen J: Bedside hemodynamic monitoring. N Engl J Med, 301:1176–1179, 1979
26. Lantiegne KC, Civetta JM: A system for maintaining invasive pressure monitoring. Heart & Lung, 7:610–621, 1978
27. Baigrie RS, Morgan CD: Hemodynamic monitoring: insertion techniques, complications and trouble-shooting. Can Med Assoc J, 121:885–892, 1979
28. Morton BC: Basic equipment requirements for hemodynamic monitoring. Can Med Assoc J, 121:879–885, 1979
29. Pugh D: Thermodilution cardiac output: What, how and why. CCQ, 2:21–28, 1979
30. Schroeder JS, Daily EK: In: Techniques in Bedside Hemodynamic monitoring. Saint Louis, CV Mosby, 1976
31. Jennings BM, Niggemann EH: Use of the balloon-tipped flow-directed catheter to assess pulmonary status. Critical Care Quarterly, 2:9–20, 1979
32. Shinn JA, Wood SL, Huseby JS: Effect of intermittent positive pressure ventilation upon pulmonary artery and pulmonary capillary wedge pressures in acutely ill patients. Heart & Lung, 8:322–327, 1979
33. Zarins CK, Virgilio RW, Smith DE, et al.: The effect of vascular volume on positive end-expiratory pressure-induced cardiac output depression and wedge-left atrial pressure discrepancy. J Surg Res, 23:348–360, 1977
34. King EG: Influence of mechanical ventilation and pulmonary disease on pulmonary pressure monitoring. Can Med Assoc J, 121:901–903, 1979
35. Berryhill RE, Benumof JL: PEEP-induced discrepancy between pulmonary arterial wedge pressure and left atrial pressure. Anesthesiology, 51:303–308, 1979
36. Giordano J, Harken A: Effect of continuous positive pressure ventilation on cardiac output. Am Surg, 41:221–224, 1975
37. Rutherford BD, McCann WP, O'Donnovan TP: The value of monitoring pulmonary artery pressure for early detection of left ventricular failure following myocardial infarction. Circulation, 43:655–665, 1971
38. Kostuk W, Barr JW, Simon AL, et al.: Correlations between the chest film and hemodynamics in acute myocardial infarction. Circulation, 48:624–632, 1973
39. Malin CG, Schwartz S: Starling curves as a guide to fluid management in the critically ill. Heart & Lung, 4:588–592, 1975
40. Dhiraj MS, Browner BD, Dutton RE, et al.: Cardiac output and pulmonary wedge pressure, use for evaluation of fluid replacement in trauma patients. Arch Surg, 112:1161–1164, 1977
41. Bland R, Shoemaker WC, Shabbot MM: Physiologic monitoring goals for the critically ill patient. Surg Gynecol Obstet, 147:833–841, 1978
42. Reininger E, Troy BL: Error in thermodilution cardiac output measurement caused by variation in syringe volume. Cathet Cardiovasc Diagn, 2:415–417, 1976
43. Buchbinder N, Ganz W: Hemodynamic monitoring: Invasive techniques. Anesthesiology, 45:146–154, 1976
44. Wallinsky P: Acute hemodynamic monitoring. Heart & Lung, 6:838–844, 1977
45. Band JD, Maki DG: Safety of changing intravenous delivery systems at longer than 24-hour intervals. Ann Intern Med, 91:173–178, 1979
46. Applefield JJ, Caruthers TE, Reno DS et al.: Assessment of sterility of long-term cardiac catheterization using the thermodilution Swan-Ganz catheter. Chest, 74:377–380, 1978
47. Weinstein RA, Stamm WE, Kramer L, et al.: Pressure monitoring devices. JAMA, 236:936–938, 1976

48. Cohn JN: Blood pressure measurement in shock: mechanism of inaccuracy in auscultory and palpatory methods. JAMA: 199:118–122, 1967
49. Berk JL: Monitoring the patient in shock. Surg Clin North Am, 55:713–720, 1975
50. Doty DB, Mosely RV: Reliable sampling of arterial blood. Surg Gynecol Obstet, 130:701–3, 1970
51. Dean WF: Surgical evaluation of volume and ventricular function. Critical Care Quarterly, 2:43–50, 1979
52. Lamb J: Intra-arterial monitoring. Nursing, 77, 7:65–71, 1977
53. Stamm WE, Colella JJ, Anderson RL, et al.: Indwelling arterial catheter as a source of nasocomial bacteremia. N Engl J Med, 292:1099–1102, 1972
54. Allen EV: Thromboangitis obliterans: Methods of diagnosis of chronic occlusive arterial lesions distal to the wrist with illustrative cases. Am J Med Sci, 178:237–44, 1929
55. Johnstone RE, Greenhow DE: Catheterization of the dorsalis pedis artery. Anesthesiology, 39:654–655, 1973
56. Nikas D, Konkoly R: Nursing responsibilities in arterial and intracranial pressure monitoring. J Neurosurg Nurs, 7:116–122, 1975
57. Gardner RM, Bond EL, Clark JS: Safety and efficacy of continuous flush systems for arterial and pulmonary artery catheters. Ann Thorac Surg, 23:531–538, 1977
58. Cole P, Simpson P, Rushman GB: Intra-arterial pressure monitoring. Anesthesiology, 31:69–72, 1976
59. Wyatt R, Glaves I, Cooper DJ: Proximal skin necrosis after radial-artery cannulation. Lancet, 1:1135–1138, 1974
60. Lowenstein E, Little JW, Lo HH: Prevention of cerebral embolization from flushing radial-artery cannulas. N Engl J Med, 285:1414–1415, 1971
61. Aubin BA: Arterial lines: A review. Critical Care Quarterly, 2:57–65, 1979
62. Downs JB, Chapman RL, Hawkins IF: Prolonged radial-artery catheterization. Arch Surg, 108:671–673, 1974
63. Bedford RF: Radial arterial function following percutaneous cannulation with 18- and 20-gauge catheters. Anesthesiology, 47:37–39, 1977

4 | Massive Blood Transfusion

Suellyn Ellerbe

The transfusion of human blood products has been part of medical practice since the early 1900s. Not until recently, however, have nurses been directly involved in blood transfusion therapy. As recently as 5 years ago in various parts of the country, nurses were not permitted to initiate blood transfusions or even to monitor the patient during transfusion therapy; these were functions of the physician.

As with other therapies that nurses have undertaken from other health professionals, the transfusion of blood and blood products may at first glance appear to be a simple technical procedure. Admittedly, the lack of formalized instruction in transfusion therapy in the undergraduate nursing curriculum, and the dearth of published information on the role of the nurse in such therapy, might contribute to the assumption that transfusion is a simple procedure.

In a study of 110 nurses practicing in a medical center in such specialty areas as trauma intensive care, the emergency room, and burn intensive care, I found that less than 40 percent understood the rationale for the various steps involved in the cross-matching and transfusion of blood. In fact, only 60 percent of the nurses studied were performing the transfusion procedure properly.[1]

Clearly, nurses have a vital role in transfusion therapy, and that role requires an understanding of the physiologic and biochemical processes affected by the collection, storage, and administration of stored blood and blood products. This chapter will review the literature pertinent to massive blood transfusion and discuss the implications of this for nursing.

BACKGROUND

With the massive-trauma casualties of the Vietnam conflict, the increasing presentation through emergency medical services of severe-trauma patients to hospital emergency rooms, and the advent of extracorporeal circulation during cardiopulmonary bypass in open-heart surgery, there has been an increasing interest in the need for providing safe methods for the administration of large quantities of banked blood. Many problems that existed in the collection, storage, and administration of banked blood in small quantities were magnified and brought into sharp focus when massive amounts of banked blood had to be administered.

It was found that the collection of blood under strict aseptic conditions in an air-free plastic container reduced the possibility of contamination by air and foreign substances.[2] Additionally the use of acid-citrate-dextrose (ACD) anticoagulant solution was found to preserve blood for up to 21 days if the blood was stored at temperatures between 1 and 6°C. When it was shown that storage of blood in citrate-phosphate-dextrose (CPD) solutions further preserves such essential components of blood as 2,3-diphosphoglyceric acid (2,3-DPG), which have profound effects on the affinity of hemoglobin for oxygen, the United States adopted the use of CPD solutions for stored blood products.

The investigation of various blood filters began when it was noted that microemboli were filtered through the pulmonary circulation, possibly contributing to the development of posttraumatic pulmonary insufficiency. The investigation led to the discovery that large amounts of debris could be transfused through the standard 170 μ filter, and that filters with pore sizes as small as 20 μ did not significantly alter blood cells, but did significantly remove from 96 to 100 percent of the debris present in stored bank blood.[3] Studies designed to elucidate the effects of administering cold bank blood versus bank blood prewarmed to body temperature (37°C) were begun when the relationship between transfusion of cold bank blood and cardiac arrhythmias became suspected. These studies showed that patients receiving large amounts of warmed blood showed significantly fewer cardiac arrhythmias produced by hypothermia than did patients receiving cold bank blood, and led to the development of effective, safe blood-warming techniques. Finally, ongoing investigation of the changes in the affinity of hemoglobin for oxygen during storage and administration of blood is leading to an increased awareness of the role of blood transfusion in restoring tissue oxygenation in critically ill patients. As a result of knowledge gained from all of the foregoing research, the administration of blood products is becoming a safer and more effective procedure.

In order to understand the implications for nursing practice surrounding massive blood transfusion, let us explore in more detail the changes that occur in blood during storage, the most important aspects in the administration of blood and blood products, and the various blood components and their indications for use.

CHANGES OCCURRING IN BLOOD DURING STORAGE

It must first be understood that blood transfusion literally constitutes tissue transplantation. Blood is a human tissue with specific antigen markings, and requires typing and crossmatching in the same way that a kidney transplant requires tissue typing and matching to prevent rejection. All too many health professionals have come to view blood transfusion therapy in the same way in which they view crystalloid intravenous therapy: that it requires some monitoring, but is basically safe and simple. This is a dangerous assumption. One reason why blood transfusion therapy is a complex and sometimes hazardous therapeutic procedure rests with the changes that occur in blood during storage, and with the implications of these changes for the nursing care of patients undergoing massive transfusion therapy.

At present, blood is collected under strictly aseptic techniques in a plastic vacuum container. An appropriate anticoagulant solution, today usually citrate-phosphate-dextrose (CPD), is added to the blood as it is collected. The blood is then stored under refrigeration, at a temperature from 1 to 6°C, until it is needed for transfusion.

Various changes occur in blood as a result of its removal from the body. These changes begin within 24 hours of storage, and continue throughout the entire 21 days of storage, after which blood is considered outdated.[2,4,5] These changes are many and varied, and probably not all of the changes in stored blood have been clearly identified.

Acid–Base Changes

Because blood is stored in an air-free container, aerobic metabolism cannot take place. However, although the hypothermic conditions under which blood is stored slow metabolism, anaerobic metabolism does occur, with the end products being lactic and pyruvic acids; thus, the longer that a given unit of blood has been in storage, the larger will be the amount of acid end products that it contains.[5] Second, the citrate used in the anticoagulant solution adds yet another acid component to banked blood. When blood is added to the CPD solution used for anticoagulation, the pH of the patient's blood immediately falls from the normal body pH of 7.4 to about 7.0. With continued red blood cell glycolysis and the accumulation of metabolic acids, the pH of CPD-treated stored blood continues to decrease to about 6.5 to 6.8 after 14 to 21 days of storage.[6] Collins, referring to the administration of large amounts of stored blood to patients in hemorrhagic hypovolemic shocks, states that:

> Both citric acid and lactic acid are normal intermediary metabolites and are rapidly metabolized under normal conditions. The pre-existing metabolic acidosis of the recipient is also an organic acidosis which is rapidly reversed when blood volume is restored, an effect that is to be

expected from the transfusion of stored blood. The impact of transfusion on the acid–base status of the recipient is, therefore, not a simple one of buffering and titration in a closed system, but rather a complex one involving rates of administration, rates of metabolic removal, and the changing circulatory efficiency of the recipient.

Alterations in Electrolyte Concentration

Because the CPD anticoagulant solution that is added to blood is a chelating agent, stored blood contains no ionized calcium. At one time, this lack of ionized calcium was considered a serious hazard, and exogenous calcium was administered periodically during massive transfusion to prevent hypocalcemia. Since most of the calcium in the body is bound to protein or stored in bone, it cannot readily be measured, thus making the diagnosis of hypocalcemia difficult and certainly impractical during massive transfusion. However, because of the lack of clinical data supporting hypocalcemia as an absolute sequel of massive transfusion, most authors now agree that the routine administration of exogenous calcium is unwise, and that patients should instead be monitored during massive transfusion for any signs and symptoms of hypocalcemia.

The sodium and potassium concentration in stored blood also undergo alteration. The absolute values of these electrolytes in stored blood vary somewhat with age, but one can expect a unit of stored blood to contain 75 to 80 mEq of sodium and 5 to 7 mEq of potassium.[6] Patients with normal cardiac and renal function appear able to handle the sodium and potassium load in stored blood even with massive blood transfusion. However, the sodium and potassium contents of stored blood may have profound effects in patients with compromised cardiac or renal function.

During blood storage there is also a progressive loss of red cell viability. Red cell organic phosphates such as adenosine triphosphate (ATP) and 2,3-diphosphoglyceric acid (2,3-DPG) become depleted.[5] The decrease in ATP produces the following changes in the red cells: (a) changes in shape from discs to spheres; (b) a loss of membrane lipid; (c) A decrease in critical hemolytic volume; and (d) a striking increase in cellular rigidity.[5,8] Along with the decrease in ATP in red cells stored at 4°C, the active transport of potassium and sodium across the cell membrane is almost halted, and the intracellular and extracellular concentrations of these two ions tend to come into equilibrium. Additionally, because of the hypotonicity of the CPD solution, red cells tend to take up water during storage.[4]

The decrease in 2,3-DPG in stored red cells produces complex changes in the affinity of hemoglobin for oxygen. Decreases in 2,3-DPG have been indicated as the cause of leftward shifts in the oxyhemoglobin dissociation curve of stored blood. Theoretically, this leftward shift could cause transfused blood cells to be less capable of releasing oxygen to the tissues than would normal blood cells.[7,9,10] However, in patients who have received massive blood transfusions, decreased levels of 2,3-DPG are not the only source of the leftward shift in the red-cell oxyhemoglobin dissociation curve; postresuscitation alkalosis and a decreased core temperature also contribute to the affinity of the red cell for oxygen. Sheldon[11] points out that following resuscitation, the combination of decreased temperature, DPG levels, and alkaline pH is associated with an increase in cardiac output, and frequently with an increase in the extraction of oxygen from blood. However, Sheldon also points out that by 24 hours after resuscitation, most patients have normal 2,3-DPG values, and that pH alterations then become the important factor in derangements of the affinity of hemoglobin for oxygen.[11] While not all of the data on the matter are yet in, it can at least be seen that there is the need for concern about the ability of stored blood to deliver oxygen to the tissues in an efficient manner.

The Microaggregate Load in Stored Blood

Another significant change that occurs in blood during storage is an increased adhesiveness and aggregation of platelets, leukocytes, and other amorphous material.[3,5,12] This causes the formation of agglomerate masses in stored blood. Practitioners have partially recognized this phenomenon for many years, and blood has been filtered through 170 μ filters to remedy it. However, electron microscope studies have now clearly identified the formation of microemboli that are considerably smaller than 170 μ.[3,12,13,14,15] Work with combat casualties during the Vietnam conflict indicated that the debris that is not trapped by an 170 μ filter is probably filtered from the circulation by the pulmonary capillary bed[3]; therefore, the administration of large quantities of blood could theoretically produce pulmonary microemboli that would lead to posttraumatic pulmonary insufficiency or the adult respiratory distress syndrome (ARDS).[3,13,15,16,17] Gervin has suggested that since platelets are

> rich sources of serotonin and other biologically active amines, these microaggregates may contain active substances which if released locally in the pulmonary vascular bed could produce significant bronchoconstriction or vasoconstriction with subsequent changes in pulmonary dynamics.

For this reason, microfilters with pore sizes ranging from 20 to 90 μ have been developed and tested. However, because the combination of shock and the various conditions requiring massive blood transfusion has been implicated in the production of ARDS, it is extremely difficult, if not impossible, to categorically prove that the use of microfilters during massive blood transfusions decreases the development of ARDS. Nevertheless, and until concrete, contrary clinical data appear, microfilters should be used when large quantities of blood are to be transfused over a short period of time, or when fewer units are being administered to patients with compromised pulmonary or cardiac status, as well as in infants and small children.[18] But whether or not the decision is made to use a microfilter during transfusion, the nurse must carefully assess the respiratory status of all patients receiving blood, and quickly report any changes in pulmonary status.

Depletion of Clotting Factors

Stored blood is deficient in most of the factors necessary for normal coagulation; it is specifically deficient in factors V, VIII, IX, and platelets. In the past, the knowledge of this led many clinicians to administer platelets and fresh frozen plasma routinely during massive transfusion. However, because the depletion of platelets and clotting factors varies widely from patient to patient, it is no longer recommended that absolute quantities of platelets and of fresh frozen plasma be administered during massive transfusion. Instead, the patient's clotting screen and bleeding status should be closely monitored during transfusion, and platelets and fresh frozen plasma should be administered only as needed (guidelines for the administration of blood components follow).

The Temperature of Stored Blood

Because blood is stored at a temperature between 1 and 6°C, it is considerably colder than human *in vivo* blood, which has a normal temperature of 37°C. It was recognized as early as 1956 that the infusion of large quantities of cold banked blood caused patients to become hypothermic, and that heart rate, blood pressure, cardiac output, and coronary blood flow fell with the decrease in body temperature that accompanied such transfusion.[14,19] The first organ to be exposed to the stream of cold banked blood is the heart. Boyan used an esophageal thermocouple placed directly behind the atria of the heart to measure temperature changes during transfusion of cold banked blood. He found marked lowering of temperature and changes in electrocardiogram tracings. The electrocardiographic alterations included marked prolongation of the S-T segment, distorted QRS complexes, peaked T waves, premature ventricular contractions, and finally bradycardia followed by cardiac standstill in two patients whose atrial temperatures had been 27.5°C and 32°C, respectively.[19] Boyan felt that these problems could be prevented by prewarming bank blood to body temperature (37°C). In a study comparing cold bank blood given to a group of 36 patients with bank blood warmed to body temperature and given to a group of 118 patients, in blood volumes of 3000 ml or more and at an infusion rate of 50 ml per minute or more, Boyan found a highly significant statistical difference in the occurrence of cardiac arrests in the two groups. Cardiac arrests occurred in 58.3 percent of the group receiving cold blood but in only 6.8 percent of the group receiving warmed blood, and this difference increased with increase in the rate and quantity of blood transfused.[19] From these studies, Boyan[19] concluded that:

> If during massive hemorrhage, an adequate blood volume is maintained by transfusing banked blood warmed to body temperature, the adverse effects of oligemia and hypothermia will be avoided.

Collins[7] points out that: "Apart from significantly increasing oxygen requirements, hypothermia interacts with many other alterations induced by massive transfusion in a detrimental way." Hypothermia impairs the metabolism of citrate and lactate, and increases the patient's risk for hypocalcemia and acidosis. Cold increases the affinity of hemoglobin for oxygen, and may impair clotting. Hypothermia also impairs the possibility of detecting a major transfusion reaction, and decreases the metabolism of anesthetic and narcotic agents.

In response to these findings, warming coils and controlled temperature baths have been developed to safely warm blood. It is important to point out that when blood is given over the normal 3 to 4 hour period, it will probably warm sufficiently to prevent complications. However, for infants and small children, patients with pretransfusion hypothermia, patients paralyzed or anesthetized or for some other reason unable to maintain their own body temperature, even a single unit of blood should probably be passed through a warming coil. And whenever one unit of blood is given in less than 3 hours, or multiple units are administered rapidly, the blood should be warmed to body temperature.

IMPORTANT PROCEDURAL ASPECTS IN THE ADMINISTRATION OF BLOOD AND BLOOD PRODUCTS

Because the administration of blood and blood products is an area in nursing practice that has very distinct legal liabilities, discussion of some of the most crucial aspects of this procedure warrant highlighting.

1. Prior to instituting blood or blood-product therapy, a physician's order must be written that clearly describes the amount of blood to be typed and crossmatched; the specific component desired; when the blood should be administered; and the period of time over which it should be administered.

2. Because of the critical consequences of administering the wrong type of blood to a patient, only the person drawing the blood or someone directly witnessing this drawing should label the blood tube. Never hand the tube to a ward secretary for labeling.

3. Blood should be maintained at a temperature of 2 to 6°C until just before transfusion. The nurse must therefore assure that blood does not stand at room temperature, is not stored in a medicine refrigerator, and is returned to the blood bank promptly if the order for transfusion is changed.

4. Blood must be inspected carefully prior to transfusion, and rejected if it has an abnormal color or appearance (for example, pink plasma, air bubbles, or a zone of hemolysis in the plasma), or if the blood bag is damaged.

5. Blood identification numbers should be checked against patient identification by two people prior to transfusion, and this cross-check should be documented on the patient's record.

6. Baseline data including vital signs, lung sounds, skin condition, urine color, and pain complaints should be collected and documented before institution of the transfusion. This permits transfusion-related changes occurring during the transfusion to be more clearly attributed to the transfusion itself.

7. Because the severity of hemolytic blood transfusion reactions is dose-dependent,[20] the nurse should remain at the patient's bedside while the first 50 cc

of blood are administered. It is also important to review the specific institution policy and procedure for administering blood and blood products, since deviation from these standards can jeopardize one legally.

BLOOD COMPONENT THERAPY

Frequently, nurses can assist physicians in selecting the appropriate components for transfusion, and in training residents in the use of blood components. This requires an understanding of the various blood components and their uses. Therefore, a brief overview of the various components follows.

Whole Blood and Packed Red Blood Cells

Although as recently as 5 years ago the question of when whole blood or packed cells should be used was controversial, virtually all authorities today agree that the only indications for the use of whole blood are when a patient is actively bleeding or has lost whole blood within the last 24 hours. In all other cases of anemia, packed red cells should be used. If flow rate becomes a problem with packed red blood cells, they may be carefully reconstituted with normal saline in the amount ordered by the physician. Occasionally, patients who have had previous transfusions or have had multiple pregnancies or abortions may develop severe, recurrent febrile reactions with the transfusion of packed red cells. In this case buffy coat-poor preparations of packed red cells may be given.

The amount of whole blood or packed red cells to be given is determined by the fact that one unit of whole blood or packed red cells can be expected to raise the hematocrit 3 percentage points. It is important to remember that children and infants have relatively smaller blood volumes than adults and, therefore, require relatively smaller "unit" sizes. In a 10 kg infant, for example, approximately 80 cc of blood can be expected to raise the hematocrit 3 percentage points.

Because they are outside the scope of this chapter, blood reactions will not be discussed in detail. However, whenever blood is ordered, the clinician must carefully weigh the significant risks involved in blood transfusions against the expected benefits. Normal hematocrit levels should probably only rarely be the goal, since no substantial evidence exists to show that moderate anemia is dangerous.

Platelets

Platelet transfusions are used in the treatment of many forms of thrombocytopenia.[21] However, because this component must be administered "fresh," the judicious use of platelets is imperative. Although some clinicians may disagree, the following recommendations are made for platelet transfusions: platelet transfusions should be considered for patients having platelet counts of less than 50,000 and who are actively bleeding, and prophylactically in patients having platelet counts of less than 20,000.[21] Platelets are stored in single units, single-donor pooled units, or multiple-donor pooled units. Rarely are single units used, but the choice of single-donor versus multiple-donor packs should be based on the amount of platelets needed, since multiple-donor packs present a higher risk of hepatitis and of alloimmunization.[21] A single unit of platelets can be expected to raise the platelet count of a 70 kg man by approximately 5,000 platelets/mm^3.

Fresh-Frozen Plasma

Fresh-frozen plasma is an essentially complete clotting package, containing all of the serum clotting factors other than platelets. Its use is primarily reserved for bleeding disorders which have not yet been delineated to a single factor, in coagulation disorders for which a single-factor preparation does not exist, and in dilutional coagulopathy associated with massive blood transfusions when alterations in clotting screens indicate the use of fresh-frozen plasma.

Cryoprecipitate and Factor IX

Cryoprecipitate is pure factor VIII; it is used in the treatment and prevention of bleeding in congenital hemophilia A and von Willebrand's disease, and in the treatment of bleeding caused by hypofribinogenemia. The amount and frequency of its administration varies with the severity of the disease.

Commercial preparations of factor IX are used specifically for the treatment of hemophilia B (Christmas disease).

Granulocytes

Despite recent advances in the collection and storage of granulocytes, their use clinically is quite circumscribed. The reason for this lies in the multiple antigenic markers present on the surface of the white blood cell, which necessitate careful histologic typing and matching, and usually limit potential donors to identical twins or close relatives. At present, granulocyte transfusion is recommended only in the treatment of leukopenia associated with neoplastic disorders when infection is present or imminent.[2]

SUMMARY

As research progresses at a rapid rate, many of the currently accepted theories and guidelines for the administration of blood and blood components and products in both routine transfusions and massive transfusions is becoming outdated. However, the foregoing discussion should provide an overview of current concepts useful in guiding the nurse in the care of patients receiving transfusions.

REFERENCES

1. Ellerbe S: An Investigation of Nurses' Practice and Knowledge in the Administration of Blood and Blood Products,'' (Master's Thesis, unpublished) Seattle, University of Washington School of Nursing, 1975
2. Heustis DW, Bove JR Busch S: Practical Blood Transfusion. Boston, Little, Brown, 1969
3. McNamara JJ, Burran EL, Suehiro G: Effective filtration of banked blood. Surgery, 71:594–597, 1972
4. American Association of Blood Banks: Technical Methods and Procedures of the American Association of Blood Banks. Chicago, Twentieth Century Press, 1980
5. Mollison PL: Blood Transfusion in Clinical Medicine. Oxford, Blackwell Scientific Publications, 1972
6. American Medical Association: General Principles of Blood Transfusion. eds. Greenwalt TJ, Polesky HF, Chaplin H, Rath CE, et al., Chicago, American Medical Association, 1977
7. Collins JA: Problems associated with the massive transfusion of stored blood. Surgery, 75:274–295, 1964
8. Longster GH, Buckley T, Sikorski J, et. al.: Scanning electron microscope studies of red cell morphology: Changes occurring in red cell shape during storage and transfusion. Vox Sang, 22:161–70, 1972
9. McConn R, Derrick JB: The respiratory function of blood: Transfusion and blood storage. Anesthesiology, 36:119–27, 1972
10. Miller RD: The oxygen dissociation curve and multiple transfusions of ACD blood. Clin Anesth, 9:41–52, 1972
11. Sheldon GF: Diphosphoglycerate in massive transfusion and erythropoiesis. Crit Care Med, 7(9):407–411, 1979
12. Ashmore PG, Swank RL, Gallery R, et al.: Effect of dacron wool filtration on the microembolic phenomenon in extracorporeal circulation. J Thorac Cardiovasc Surg, 63:240–248, 1972
13. Gervin AS, Mason KG, Wright CB: Ultrapore hemofiltration: The effects on the coagulation and fibrinolytic mechanisms in fresh and stored blood. Arch Surg, 106:333–336, 1973
14. Goldiner PL: New concepts in the administration of bank blood. Clin Anesth, 9:51–67, 1972
15. Reul GJ Jr, Greenberg DS, Lefrak EA, et al.: Prevention of post-traumatic pulmonary insufficiency: Fine screen filtration of blood. Arch Surg, 106:386–394, 1973
16. Blaisdell WF, Schlobohm, RM: The respiratory distress syndrome: A review. Surgery, 74:251–262, 1973
17. Shires GT, Carrico CJ, Canizaro PC: Shock. Philadelphia, WB Saunders, 1973
18. International Forum: Does a relationship exist between massive blood transfusion and the adult respiratory distress syndrome? Vox Sang, 32(5):311–320, 1977
19. Boyan CP: Cold or warmed blood for massive transfusion. Ann Surg, 160:282–286, 1964
20. Goldfinger D: Acute hemolytic transfusion reactions. Transfusion, 17(2):85–98, 1977
21. Aisner J: Platelet transfusion therapy. Med Clin North Am, 61(5):1133–45, 1977
22. Schiffer CA: Principles of Granulocyte Transfusion Therapy. Med Clin North Am, 61(5):1119–1131, 1977

SUGGESTED READINGS

Dybkjaer E, Elkjaer P: The use of heated blood in massive blood replacement. Acta Anesthesiol Scand, 8:271–278, 1964

Gervin AS, Mason KG, Wright CB: Micro-aggregate volumes in stored human blood. Surg Gynecol Obstet, 139:519–524, 1974

Guyton AC: Basic Human Physiology: Normal Function and Mechanisms of Disease. Philadelphia, WB Saunders, 1971

Hinkes E, Steffen RO: Current transfusion therapy. Calif Med, 118:38–55, 1973

Miller RD: Complications of Massive Blood Transfusions. Anesthesiology, 39:82–92, 1973

Schmidt PJ: Regulatory transfusion therapy. Ann Clin Lab Sci, 3:305–306, 1973

Schmidt PJ: Safe and effective transfusions. Prog Clin Pathol, 2:168–197, 1969

Valeri CR, Bryan-Brown CW, Altschule M: (guest eds.), Symposium on function of red blood cells. Crit Care Med, 7(9):407–411, 1979.

Westphal RG: Rational alternatives to the use of whole blood. Ann. Intern Med, 76:987–990, 1972

Wilson RF, Gibson D, Percinel AK, et al.: Eight years of experience with massive blood transfusions. J Trauma, 11:275–285, 1971

5 | Colloid Versus Crystalloid Fluid Resuscitation in Shock and Injury

John T. Corpening

The effective clinical management of the severely injured patient with hemorrhage accompanied by shock requires an organized approach to insure the rapid establishment and maintenance of an airway, fluid volume replacement, and the control of hemorrhage. The immediate restoration of an effective circulating blood volume through use of a balanced salt solution, colloid solution, or both, the institution of therapies to minimize or reverse the biochemical sequelae of shock, and rapid surgical intervention as needed have significantly reduced the use of uncrossmatched blood. This approach has reduced the mortality rates and decreased the incidence of complications in low flow states. However, the prevailing concepts of fluid resuscitation are currently represented by two schools of thought. Each of these schools will be examined by exploring their respective supporting data. The objective is not to conclude with a judgement, but rather to elucidate for the clinician the current theories surrounding fluid resuscitation.

THE CRYSTALLOID SCHOOL

In the late 1930s and early 1940s, Blalock first described the distributional changes in body fluids following injury.[1] Later, Moyer reported the contribution

61

of the interstitial fluid to these posttraumatic distributional changes.[2] Initially, these changes do not result in electrolyte concentration changes, since they occur in an isotonic manner; the event precipitating eventual changes in electrolyte concentrations is a loss of extracellular fluid (ECF). A major function of ECF is the transport of nutrients between the vasculature and the cells, and substantial losses (or distributional changes) of ECF result in impairment of this vital function. Consequently, with ECF loss, cellular processes are significantly impaired despite adequate intravascular volume replacement. Therefore, ECF replacement is essential to the restoration of cellular function—which is a direct correlate of patient survival.

ECF loss may occur in one of three ways:

1.   Absolute loss, through diarrhea, vomiting, gastrointestinal suction, and fistula drainage.
2.   "Third-space loss" (distributional shift), through soft-tissue injuries, fractures, and ascites.
3.   Intracellular loss, through distributional change accompanying hemorrhagic shock.

Shires' data have demonstrated that hemorrhagic shock is accompanied by a loss of ECF that is greater than could be accounted for by the volume of blood lost alone.[3] His extensive investigation, utilizing tracer dilution curves in both treated and untreated hemorrhagic shock, demonstrated a reduction in the total ECF volume when compared with the control value. One explanation for the decrease in ECF volume in untreated hemorrhagic shock is that interstitial fluid moves into cells in an isotonic fashion.

Shires also studied ion transport across cell membranes to determine whether intracellular swelling took place in response to hemorrhagic shock. In Shires' initial studies, ultramicroelectrodes recorded transmembrane potentials (PD) in hemorrhagic preparations (mice). As expected, the resting PD in prehemorrhagic preparations was -90 mv. When the prepared animals were subjected to hemorrhage, the decrease in blood pressure was closely paralleled by a decrease in PD, until a plateau was reached at -60 mv. Studies were then done to determine whether the decrease in PD in hemorrhagic shock was dependent on changes in ECF composition. Shires' data demonstrated that the PD was independent of changes in pH, pCO_2, HCO_3^- concentration, or serum potassium levels. In that the PD showed a close correlation with the decrease in blood pressure, it appears that the decrease in PD is secondary to hypoperfusion. Briefly, the change in cell membrane potential in hemorrhagic shock may be due to either (a) inhibition of membrane ion pumping, or (b) a selective increase in cell membrane permeability to sodium. Further studies by Shires, on subhuman primates, resulted in identical findings[4]; PD in hemorrhagic subjects (baboons) fell to -60 mv. When the subjects were resuscitated with balanced salt solution (lactated Ringer's solution), however, the membrane potential rose to normal levels. There was no significant change in the total water content of biopsied muscles in the preshock and shock states. A 49 percent decrease in extracellular water (ECW) was observed, however, accompanied by a 6 percent increase in intracellular water (ICW). The following changes in the electrolyte composition of the biopsied tissue were noted:

1. An increase in the ICW sodium from 9.9 mEq/L to 18.4 mEq/L (+85 percent) in the shock state.
2. A 185 percent increase in ICW chloride in the shock state.
3. A 118 percent increase in extracellular potassium in the shock state.

A significant point in Shires' results is that the intracellular redistribution of ions following prolonged shock was not accompanied by a change in the total electrolyte content of the tissue studied (skeletal muscle). In explanation of Shires' findings, I propose the algorithm set out in Figure 5-1.

The crystalloid school, therefore, advocates the use of balanced salt solution (lactated Ringer's solution) as the mechanism for restoring ECF volume and decreasing mortality and morbidity[5] from shock due to injury. It should be noted that whole blood is used to replace cell mass when the hematocrit falls below 30 percent. In the few cases of extreme blood loss, type-specific whole blood (which can be made available within 10 to 15 minutes after admission) is used. In the rare instance of exsanguinating hemorrhage (from a ruptured aorta, a heart wound, or other massive vascular injury), administration of O-negative blood is begun as soon as possible.

In cases in which blood is required to replace cell mass, concurrent alleviation of the reduction in functional ECF volume is desirable. Lactated Ringer's solution, as previously mentioned, is the advocated therapeutic adjunct. Lactated Ringer's solution is isotonic, essentially free from side effects, and harmless from the standpoint of aggravation of other fluid and electrolyte imbalances that may be present. Additionally, the use of blood plus lactated Ringer's solution results in a more rapid return to normal of lactate levels and pH than does treatment with blood alone.[6]

The rapid restoration of ECF volume deficits and the restoration of blood flow have eliminated oliguric renal failure as a complication of shock. The crystalloid school does not advocate the use of plasma or albumin as volume expanders. Moore estimates that plasma dispersal from the intravascular to the extravascular compartment may proceed at a rate approaching 500 ml (two units) per hour.[7] Therefore, plasma or albumin as blood-volume substitutes have only transient effects at best. However, if whole blood is unavailable and will not be available within a reasonable period, plasma or 5 percent albumin solution, administered as stop-gap measures, is probably reasonable after replacement of ECF deficits with balanced salt solution.

THE COLLOID SCHOOL

The colloid school of thought, as opposed to the crystalloid, holds that the primary problem in acute circulatory failure is the restoration of plasma volume,

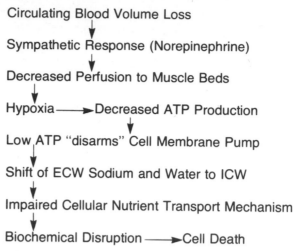

Fig. 5-1. Biochemical sequence in shock

and therefore of oxygen transport. According to this philosophy, hemodynamic stability is achieved with normal or supernormal blood volumes providing the adequate oxygen and nutrients needed for the restoration of cellular function. Inadequate circulatory blood volume, owing to hemorrhage or redistribution of the normal blood volume by pooling in the microcirculation, causes a marked decrease in venous return, and therefore a diminished cardiac output. Shoemaker's data demonstrated, through a variety of cardiorespiratory parameters, that—in order to meet the increased metabolic needs associated with tissue repair and fever[8]—survivors of shock required blood volumes approximately 500 ml in excess of normal, predicted values. The increased plasma volume and cardiac index produced by colloid administration were associated with improved oxygen availability and oxygen consumption ($\overset{\circ}{V}O_2$). This appears to suggest that the improved hemodynamics associated with the administration of colloids led to improved tissue perfusion.

A decreased $\overset{\circ}{V}O_2$ has been documented as the common major and critical physiologic problem in the early stages of various types of shock.[9] Therefore, in resuscitation, it is necessary to restore the $\overset{\circ}{V}O_2$ not simply to its normal values, but to optimal values. Shoemaker argues that the ability of an agent to restore the $\overset{\circ}{V}O_2$ to normal values may be the best measure of its effectiveness. In his studies, dextran-40 was the most potent plasma expander. With use of this agent, oxygen consumption averaged 43 ± 8 ml/min/m², which was better than the oxygen consumption value following the administration of whole blood (33 ± 6 ml/min/m²) or 5 percent albumin (35 ± 9 ml/min/m²). There were no significant $\overset{\circ}{V}O_2$ changes following the administration of crystalloid. The colloid school also argues that irrespective of how and why sodium leaks into cells during shock, the restoration of normal cellular function requires the action of the energy-dependent (ATP) sodium pump, and not the addition of sodium.

If crystalloids are used as the primary resuscitative agents following shock, the volumes required to achieve normal hemodynamic values are from two to four times those required with colloids. Furthermore, massive crystalloid fluid resuscitation predisposes the patient to the adult respiratory distress syndrome (ARDS), a subject addressed at length in this book. As an added point, the colloid school argues that the amount of colloid "leak" into the interstitial lung space is negligible compared with that of crystalloid.[10,11]

NEWER DEVELOPMENTS

School arguments aside, more recent research appears to indicate that albumin does expose the patient to a greater risk of pulmonary insufficiency and ARDS than originally postulated.[12] Lucas and co-workers at Detroit General Hospital were well aware of the controversy surrounding the ideal fluid resuscitative regimen of the injured patient in shock; at that institution, colloids and crystalloids were administered according to availability and personal preference—a situation probably not unique. In controlled studies of 94 patients, Lucas' group found that those who received colloids as their primary resuscitative fluid had a 10 percent greater pulmonary shunt and required ventilatory support for 5 days longer than did patients who received crystalloids. Their data appear to confirm that the addition of supplemental albumin to standard resuscitation regimens for hypovolemic shock due to injury worsens pulmonary function.

Considerable controversy continues to surround the choice of fluids for resuscitation from shock and injury states, as well as the choice of fluids for the care of the critically ill patient with multiple organ system failure. Each of the fluids available for such application has both advantages and disadvantages.

1.   Whole blood and red blood cells are limited by cost, availability, risk of hepatitis, and the time needed for crossmatching.
2.   Crystalloids are advocated for filling the ECF, but usually expand the interstitial space as well, particularly in the lung.
3.   Colloids restore plasma volume without producing water overload, but have recently been implicated in respiratory insufficiency.

In the initial fluid resuscitation from shock and injury, the primary objective is to achieve hemodynamic stability through volume therapy that produces ECF-volume, blood-flow, and oxygen-consumption values that vary from acceptable to optimal. Regardless of the agent or combination of agents chosen, it is imperative that the patient's cardiopulmonary dynamics be monitored in such a way that reliable physiologic trends and responses to therapy can be established. Parameters used to establish a baseline and to provide ongoing monitoring include:

1.   Blood pressure and pulse rate.
2.   Pulmonary artery wedge pressure.
3.   Cardiac output and index.

BACKGROUND

Put simply, the GI tract extends from the mouth to the anus. Numerous authors quibble about the length of the tract, setting this at from 20 to 28 feet. Few argue its divisions which, for the most part, can be classified into an upper gastrointestinal tract, extending from the mouth to the ileocecal valve, and a lower gastrointestinal tract, extending from the ileocecal valve to the anus. Once clearly envisioned, it can be seen that the human is, in fact, a being centered around a tube that is essentially continuous with the environment. From this tube all fluid and nutrients in the healthy human are absorbed, and those dietary byproducts and unusable fluids and electrolytes not needed by the body are expelled.

The gastrointestinal tract itself, then, accomplishes two major functions in the maintenance of homeostasis: (a) digestion and (b) absorption. Digestion is the preparation of ingested food and foodstuffs for use by the body; it is thus the mechanical aspect of survival, and involves such activities as mastication, swallowing, appropriate rates of gastric motility, and the secretion of various substances. These activities ultimately reduce large and compound substances to minute and often discrete molecular components in preparation for absorption. Absorption, on the other hand, is the actual movement of the products of digestion from the enteral tube to the internal environment of the cell. Here the various absorbed substances become the supporting elements in optimum bodily and mental function. Thus, absorption is the synthesizing aspect of the gastrointestinal system and involves such facets as diffusion, active transport, and recombination.

However, although digestion and absorption can be spoken of separately for the sake of theoretical understanding, this approach should not be confused with the reality present in the functioning gastrointestinal tract. Digestion and absorption occur simultaneously, and although certain functions can be attributed more to one than to the other, many of the functions of both overlap and are essential to the transport of fluid and nutrients from the external to the internal environment. (The sites of absorption of major nutrients are presented in Figure 6-1 and the composition of the fasting GI tract in Figure 6-2).

The fluid and nutritional requirements necessary for maintenance of homeostasis vary according to age, sex, body build, state of health, and activity level. Generally speaking, however, the fluid requirements of the average active adult are from 2 to 3 L/24 hours.[1,2,3] The caloric requirements for this same individual would range from 2,000 to 5,000 calories/24 hours for maintenance of the body in a steady state, with neither loss nor gain of weight.[4] Numerous stress factors can add to both the fluid and caloric requirements of the hospitalized patient. Some classic examples are elevated temperature, surgical intervention, burns, and loss of significant body fluids—particularly protein, as from fistulae.[5,6,7]

Finally, it is becoming increasingly apparent that vitamins and minerals are necessary for the promotion of health and the maintenance of homeostasis. Some key examples are thiamine (vitamin B_1), which is essential for the oxida-

SITES OF ABSORPTION

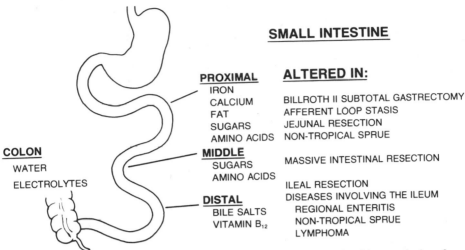

SMALL INTESTINE

PROXIMAL
IRON
CALCIUM
FAT
SUGARS
AMINO ACIDS

MIDDLE
SUGARS
AMINO ACIDS

DISTAL
BILE SALTS
VITAMIN B$_{12}$

COLON
WATER
ELECTROLYTES

ALTERED IN:

BILLROTH II SUBTOTAL GASTRECTOMY
AFFERENT LOOP STASIS
JEJUNAL RESECTION
NON-TROPICAL SPRUE

MASSIVE INTESTINAL RESECTION

ILEAL RESECTION
DISEASES INVOLVING THE ILEUM
    REGIONAL ENTERITIS
    NON-TROPICAL SPRUE
    LYMPHOMA

Fig. 6-1. Sites of absorption of major nutrients (Reproduced with permission from Greenberger NJ, Winship DH: Gastrointestinal Disorders: A Pathophysiologic Approach. Copyright © 1976 by Year Book Medical Publishers, Inc., Chicago. p. 115.)

tion of carbohydrates and the maintenance of normal gastrointestinal activity. Often, vitamin B deficiencies are present in the patient with chronic gastrointestinal disease. Vitamins C and K are two other examples of key elements that can become deficient in the patient with a gastrointestinal disorder.[8,9]

Because it would be beyond the scope of this chapter to describe all of the possible interruptions or alterations, or both, of the GI tract that affect fluid management, three key examples have been selected. In many ways these conditions, once understood, act as prototypes for the management of other conditions. The three conditions to be discussed are vomiting or continuous nasogastric suction, small bowel fistulae, and diarrhea.

VOMITING OR CONTINUOUS NASOGASTRIC SUCTION

Vomiting occurs in numerous situations and can be caused by factors as varied as pregnancy or duodenal obstruction. In most cases it represents a transient condition that requires little more than brief cessation of food and fluid intake, accompanied by rest. However, in the event of pyloric obstruction, vomiting may be accompanied by pronounced peristaltic waves observable on the abdominal wall. Often the vomitus will contain particles of food from a previous meal in addition to the fluid lost. If bleeding has occurred in the upper GI tract, the acid environment of the stomach causes the vomitus to assume a brown tone. The vomiting of fecal contents or foul-smelling emesis obviously indicates a small intestinal obstruction or lower GI occlusion. The presence of bile in the vomitus usually indicates an obstruction distal to the pyloric sphincter.

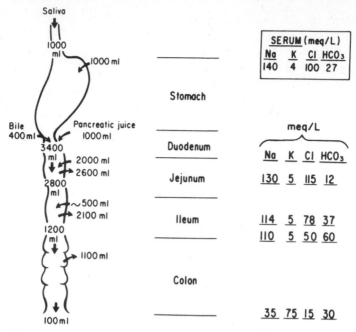

Fig. 6-2.   Secretion, absorption, intraluminal flow rate (ml/day) and composition of fasting gastrointestinal tract contents in man (From: Frohlich ED, ed.: Pathophysiology: Altered Regulatory Mechanisms in Disease, 2nd edn. Philadelphia, JB Lippincott, 1976, p. 509.)

The more distal the obstruction of the GI tract, the more delayed (if not altogether absent) will be the vomiting. With obstruction in the upper GI tract, however, the onset of vomiting can be rapid and severe, and water and electrolyte losses can quickly become acute. Because of this, prolonged vomiting or high-output nasogastric suctioning can progress from the symptom of an illness to a condition which in and of itself requires aggressive treatment. [10,11]

Although the normal stomach and upper GI contents total approximately 2,500 ml, progressive and continuous vomiting or suctioning can produce large alterations in body fluids, with losses ranging from 100 to 1,600 ml in 24 hours. Furthermore, because gastric secretions contain sodium (Na^+), potassium (K^+), and hydrochloric acid (HCl), continuous vomiting can and does represent the threat of saline depletion, and ultimately affects the volume of the extracellular space. The increased loss of K^+ and HCl can rapidly affect the pH of the body, and ultimately put the patient in metabolic alkalosis. If lost K^+ is not replaced, hypokalemia ensues with its major effect of muscular weakness; all major muscles including the cardiac, skeletal, respiratory, and intestinal groups are affected.

Generally speaking, excessive vomiting or continuous upper GI suctioning, left untreated, results in fluid volume depletion, metabolic alkalosis, potassium deficit, and sodium loss. When loss of upper gastric secretions becomes excessive, it most frequently is the result of upper GI obstruction, gastroenteritis, acute pancreatitis, or a common-duct stone[12]; the symptoms can be expected to subside if the obstruction is removed, a procedure often involving surgical intervention. Prior to removal of the obstruction by whatever means, it becomes imperative to treat the symptoms by (a) making the vomiting subside, usually by administering antiemetics; and (b) by replacing fluids and electrolytes adequately by the parental route. In either approach, the patient should receive nothing by mouth. Gastric secretions are greatly reduced when the stomach is at rest. The cessation of food or fluids by mouth is often adequate therapy in and of itself.[1]

In either prolonged vomiting or continuous suctioning, accurate recording of type and amount of secretion should be made by the nurse. Because of the tonicity of GI secretions, the fluid used to replace that which has been lost should contain some percentage of sodium chloride, with consideration given to concurrent medical problems such as right heart failure or renal disease. Additionally, appropriate electrolytes should be added to replace the K^+ and chloride (Cl^-) lost. Replacement should be calculated according to the quantities of electrolytes in the secretions being lost, as well as the pH of these secretions. Unless K^+ deficit is severe (less than 3 mEq/L), replacement of K^+ in particular should be carried out at a rate of no more than 20 mEq/hour.[2,3,13]

If irrigation of nasogastric tubes is necessary, the nurse should irrigate with 30 to 50 ml of air or use isotonic saline so as to avoid further loss of electrolytes via suctioning. If ice chips are given to the patient, they too should be made from saline and not water. In all, comfort should be provided the patient in order to reduce stimuli and the number of irritants in the environment should be controlled.[1,3,13]

In many cases the duration of vomiting or suctioning is not extensive enough to warrant replacement of large numbers of calories. Dietary intake when resumed, however, should progress slowly and only after the cause of vomiting has been removed and obvious signs of peristalsis have returned such as the passing of flatus, hunger, and the presence of bowel sounds.

FISTULAE

Perhaps one of the most serious and potentially life-threatening situations in terms of GI disease occurs with the presentation of one or more small-bowel fistulae. In order to approach such patients, one must have a thorough understanding of the portion of the bowel affected. Moreover, it is imperative that the normal amount, quality, and composition of the secretions characteristic of the affected portion of the GI tract be understood. A review of the amounts of GI secretions and their electrolyte contents appears in Table 1-1 and Figure 1-1 (see Chapter 1).

An external fistula is a tubelike structure, with openings at each end, which forms a hollow tract between an injured part of the bowel and the external environment. In all cases the result of the formation of this passageway is the excretion of secretions that are normally routed internally through the GI tract. The fistula may form spontaneously, as the result of disease, but approximately

95 percent of such fistulae are complications of surgical procedures, as in the case of anastomotic dehiscence or injury to the bowel during dissection. Fistulae are also prone to develop following the removal of adhesions or as a result of inflamed intestines or radiation enteropathy. Frequently these fistulae are accompanied by abscesses and are therefore often preceded by fever and abdominal pain.[14]

Next to the development of sepsis, perhaps the greatest potentially life-threatening complication occurring in the patient with small-bowel fistulae is the excessive loss of both fluid and electrolytes. A review of Figures 6-1 and 6-2 reminds one of the magnitude of potential fluid and electrolyte losses in such cases. If these losses are not reversed, dehydration and malnutrition ensues, followed by sepsis, multiple organ failure, and death.

Because the secretions in the small bowel are both isotonic and hypertonic, loss of secretions via a fistula requires their replacement in the same quantity and type of solution in order to maintain the volume in the vascular space and ultimately the total body water. This is usually accomplished by administering isotonic saline milliliter for milliliter for the quantity of fluid lost. Insensible losses and daily basic fluid requirements are met with additional hypotonic fluids as warranted, throughout the course of therapy.

Simultaneous with the replacement of fluid is the collection of the secretions being expelled from the fistula(e) itself. This not only provides for the accurate calculation of fluid replacement needs, but also allows for secretions, along with urinary output, to be sent to the laboratory for electrolyte content analysis. With this data in hand, one can select replacement fluids that are appropriate to the fluid being lost.

Owing to the presence of large amounts of digestive enzymes in the small bowel, it becomes essential that fistula secretions not come in contact with the skin. If the fistula is left to drain freely, excoriation and skin breakdown inevitably result. This is a complication no longer excusable in this day of multiple appliances and adhesives.[3,15]

For the most acute losses occurring in both large and small-bowel fistulae, restoration of normal vascular volume and electrolyte concentration is usually accomplished within hours to days. Following this replacement, the patient's nutritional needs must be addressed. Given an understanding that in healthy humans the great preponderance of absorption of nutrients occurs in the small intestine, it is obvious that one or more fistula(e) can result in rapid nutritional depletion. Accompanying this depletion are weight loss due to a catabolic state, poor wound and skin healing, weakness, decreased mentation, and other complications. In the past, for the patient with a fistula, these sequelae were common, since the only available source of nutrition for these patients was the standard 5 percent dextrose intravenous solution, which, given at a rate of 125 cc per hour, provides approximately 700 kcal in 24 hours, whereas the fistula patient frequently requires 3,000 kcal/24 hours. Indeed, according to the amount and type of secretions lost, the presence of elevated temperature, recent surgical wounds, infection or sepsis, and the level of physical activity, the fistula patient may require upwards of 6,000 kcal/24 hours. Obviously, needs of this magnitude cannot be met with the standard 5 percent dextrose solution. Today, there are two primary methods for providing the calories and nutrients required by these patients: (a) enteral feedings; and (b) total parenteral nutrition (TPN), or hyperalimentation.

Enteral Feedings

Enteral feedings are a source of nutrition in liquid form which can be ingested orally or through a nasogastric or nasoduodenal tube. Although first used by Rose in 1940, advances have been made in recent years in the preparation of these mixtures, and there are now various brands available that provide specific nutrients to different types of patients with GI conditions ranging from pancreatic insufficiency to radiation enteritis.[16,17,18]

The enteral form of nutrient source is usually not used in the early stages of fistula management, for although such feeding could probably provide some calories, the position of the small-bowel fistula usually excludes this as a viable therapeutic modality. If the fistula is distal to the stomach or duodenum, most of the feeding, by whatever route administered, is lost to the GI system, which only further compounds the problem; the accurate calculation of both fistula(e) output and caloric availability would then become impossible. Finally, owing to the fact that enteral feedings are received into the upper GI tract, peristalsis and enzyme secretions would ensue, defeating the goal of reducing fistula output and maintaining a quiet bowel. In the case of low-output fistulae, it is suggested that enteral feeding be used, and that a central line be inserted for the simultaneous administration of hyperalimentation.

Total Parenteral Nutrition

In 1968, Dudrick and his associates developed a method of supplying total parenteral nutrition (TPN) to the patient for whom other methods of nutritional support were impossible. Prior to this, patients with GI disorders suffered a 50 percent mortality rate; particularly was this so among patients with enterocutaneous fistulae, and even more specifically among patients with duodenal or jejunal fistula(e). Recently, with the availability of TPN, these figures have been reversed. Reports indicate that spontaneous closure rates of these types of fistulae may be as high as 50 to 70 percent when patients with such fistulae are treated with hyperalimentation and a positive nitrogen balance is achieved.[19,20]

"Parenteral hyperalimentation," states Borgen, "is the intravenous delivery of essential nutrients to maintain a patient in positive nitrogen balance and nutritional equilibrium. It is indicated when gastrointestinal intake is impossible, potentially hazardous or insufficient."[21] Because of the hypertonic dextrose made available by these solutions, large amounts of calories can be supplied. Other than hypertonic dextrose, the solutions usually contain amino acids, electrolytes, vitamins, and trace elements. Simply stated, the amino acids provide the nitrogen source in TPN, while the hypertonic dextrose provides the calories.

When possible, fat emulsions can and should be administered with parenteral hyperalimentation as an additional source of calories (9 kcal/g). Because fat emulsions are isotonic they may be administered peripherally, and are thus not accompanied by the potentially hazardous side-effects inherent with a central line. However, use of emulsions is contraindicated in patients with fat metabolism disorders, such as pathogenic hyperlipidemia or acute pancreatitis with hyperlipidemia, severe liver damage, or threatened fat embolism. Nor should these solutions be mixed with any other solutions, or any electrolytes, drugs or vitamins be added to them.[22]

Because the general approach to the treatment of any patient who is to be placed on TPN is covered by numerous authors,[8,21,23] it will not be repeated here. However, due to the fact that patients with enterocutaneous fistulae suffer concurrent fluid, electrolyte, and plasma protein losses, several points particular to these patients will be made.

Because of the loss of large amounts of electrolytes from the small bowel—particularly Na^+ and K^+, it is necessary for the nurse to pay close attention to the serum Na^+ and serum K^+ levels. Maintenance of both of these electrolytes within normal limits is essential to insure appropriate cellular function, and additionally to allow for the transmission of nutrients into the cell via the "carrier function." With the infusion of hypertonic glucose, the serum insulin level is elevated, causing an increased influx of K^+ and glucose into the cell. Therefore, although normal K^+ requirements are 30 to 50 mEq/day, the potassium requirements of a patient on TPN may rise to as high as 80 to 120 mEq (with the administration of 4,000 kcal/24 hours). As a general rule, 40 mEq of K^+ should be administered per 1,000 kcal given. In certain conditions where K^+ loss is elevated and absorption in the intestinal tract is decreased, as in GI fistulae, additional K^+ has to be supplied, so long as renal function is satisfactory.

In the early stages of fistula management, bed rest is often a reality. Because of this, calcium leaves the skeleton and enters the blood stream, and this increased serum calcium, particularly in the presence of decreased total body water and alkaline urine, may cause stone formation. The administration of magnesium appears to protect against such stone formation, and for this reason, and because it is present in the GI tract, magnesium is another necessary component of hyperalimentation therapy.

The small intestine is generally an alkaline environment. Increased fluid loss via fistula(e) drainage causes the loss of bicarbonate (HCO_3^-) and the concurrent retention of increased quantities of Cl^-. Left untreated, this situation will result in metabolic acidosis; shortness of breath progressing to weakness and generalized malaise can become the visible sign of this condition. The HCO_3^- loss in fistula drainage must therefore be given special attention in the selection of appropriate amounts of additives to the basic TPN solution.

Because some of the vitamins essential to the utilization of nutrients are stored in small amounts in the body, it is vital that their addition to the hypertonic solution become an integral part of the treatment of patients receiving TPN. The necessity of selected vitamins in treatment grows in importance the longer the patient remains on hyperalimentation. Furthermore, the role of vitamins in relation to the patient's ability to handle stress is now receiving increased attention. The fistula patient presents the health care team with a classic picture of physiologic and psychologic stress. In order to address these stress and nutritional needs, vitamins C and B complex are routinely administered. If the patient remains on TPN for extended periods, it may become necessary to also provide the fat-soluble vitamins A and D; however, in many cases, because the length of time on that the patient receives TPN is not excessive, this is unnecessary.

Nurses often react to the seeming megadose quantities of vitamins ordered for TPN patients. This approach is deliberate, in order to: (a) provide for increased vitamin demand, as in the demand for vitamin C, with its role in wound healing; and (b) compensate for vitamin losses through urinary excretion. In the fistula patient, vitamin B is of particular importance for its role in assisting carbohydrate metabolism and in maintaining normal GI function. Vitamin therapy should be spread over the full 24 hour period of the day in order to assure better vitamin utilization. Usually, vitamins B_{12}, K, and folic acid are given intramuscularly, intermittently, and only to patients who are on TPN for prolonged periods. In most cases, it is unnecessary to provide iron via the parenteral route unless preexisting conditions, such as previous hemorrhage, warrant it. The trace elements of zinc, copper, manganese, cobalt, and iodine are becoming a standard part of therapy for all patients receiving hyperalimentation.[24]

It is impossible to put sufficient emphasis on the importance of maintaining strict sterile technique in the changing of hyperalimentation dressings, and on the need for close monitoring of the patient receiving hyperalimentation solutions. In some cases, as the use of TPN becomes more common, its hazards and potentially life-threatening consequences to the patient are viewed less seriously. Hospital protocols should be clearly established and adhered to by all staff, and the physiologic effects of delivering hyperosmolar solutions should be reviewed by the hospital staff at regular intervals.

Although for some fistula patients activity in the early stages of treatment is somewhat restricted owing to the quantities of secretions, planned activity, exercise, or both is necessary for the proper use of available nutrients. For classical reasons, all patients should exercise, but the patient on TPN defeats the purpose of his or her treatment if left on bed rest without exercise. The reason for this lies in the increased amount of nitrogen excreted by the immobile patient. Exercise decreases this urinary nitrogen loss and restores a positive nitrogen balance more quickly.[9]

Finally, some patients with small bowel fistulae receive cimetidine (Tagamet). This drug, a histamine H_2-receptor blocking agent, acts to reduce gastric acid secretion and in some cases actually reduces fistula output, thus accomplishing one of the goals of fistula therapy.[14]

The treatment of small-bowel fistulae has been radically improved since total parenteral nutrition has become available. The approach to the patient with such fistulae is rather direct, comprising (a) restoration of volume and replacement of fluid and electrolyte losses; (b) drainage of abscesses; (c) control of the fistula drainage and recording of its output; (d) provision of intravenous therapy;

(e) maintenance of a caloric intake of 3,000 kcal or more per day; and (f) preparation of the patient for surgery if the fistula(e) fail to close.[14]

DIARRHEA

Diarrhea, say several authors, is the increased fecal loss of water and electrolytes. It is characterized by a stool weight of greater than 200 g and by an increased frequency of defecation. Since all stool weight is approximately 80 percent water, it follows that any increased stool weight is caused by an increase in stool water.[10,25]

The causes of diarrhea can be vast, and can range from something as transient as a brief response to a cathartic to the prolonged and debilitating diarrhea of Crohn's disease.

For the most part, the fluid and electrolytes lost via diarrhea are similar to those covered in the discussion of small bowel fistula. However, the quantities of electrolytes in the stool in diarrhea are lower. As the stool volume—which can reach as high as 17,000 ml/24 hours—increases, Na^+ loss increases, and K^+ loss decreases. Because of the high concentration of HCO_3^- in the lower bowel, diarrhea can lead to metabolic acidosis. And if not reversed promptly, diarrhea can easily result in water and electrolyte depletion, weight loss, malaise, and deficiencies in vitamins and minerals, as well as serious alterations in acid–base balance.

The treatment of diarrhea revolves around clearly delineating its etiology, while at the same time aggressively treating its symptoms. With respect to the latter, both isotonic and hypotonic solutions should be given. Intake and output, as well as specific gravity and blood pressure should be strictly and frequently monitored until stabilization occurs. Frequently stool samples should be collected for laboratory analysis.

Once fluid volume has been restored, it becomes the task of the health care team to either further delineate the problem in any specific case of diarrhea or, if the latter has been identified, to plan specific treatment. In most cases of severe diarrhea, a period of time to allow the bowel to rest is warranted. During this interval, calories should be given in some form; hyperalimenation may be the treatment form of choice. In certain situations prolonged diarrhea or the inability to absorb nutrients may require the placement of a Broviac catheter for long-term TPN. In any event, the goal of the health care team in the treatment of severe diarrhea is (a) replacement of fluids and electrolytes, (b) administration of a caloric substance, and (c) identification of the etiology of the diarrhea.

SUMMARY

Gastrointestinal physiology, even in its normal state, presents the health care worker with a vast area of study. Alterations in GI physiology affect not only the fluid, electrolyte, and nutritional status of the system itself, but ultimately also influence the environment of every cell within the organism. With increased knowledge and new care techniques there has arisen a healthy respect for the key role of the GI tract in homeostasis. Nurses have a significant part in monitoring this system. Ultimately, their awareness, knowledge, suggestions for treatment, and evaluation of therapeutic regimens will influence the well-being of the patient—and most particularly of the critically ill patient.

REFERENCES

1. Metheny N, Snively W: Nurses' Handbook of Fluid Balance, 2nd edn. Philadelphia, JB Lippincott, 1974
2. Dressler D: Homeostasis: The balanced state. In: Monitoring Fluid and Electrolytes Precisely. Horsham, PA, Nursing '78 Books, Intermed Communications, 1978
3. Given B, Simmons S: Gastroenterology in Clinical Nursing. St. Louis, CV Mosby, 1975
4. Guyton A: Texbook of Medical Physiology, 5th edn. Philadelphia, WB Saunders, 1976
5. Butterworth C: The skeleton in the hospital closet. Nutrition Today 9(2): 4–8, 1974
6. Hill G: Surgical Malnutrition, Nursing Mirror 145(20): 17–19, 1977
7. Donovan L: Is the doctor starving your patient? RN 41(7): 36–40, 1978
8. Walike B: Disturbances of Food Intake and Nutrition. In: Nursing Care of the Patient with Medical-Surgical Disorders, 2nd edn., eds. Moidel H, Giblin E, Wagner B. New York, McGraw-Hill, pp. 251–270, 1971
9. Levenson S, Seifter E, Van Winkle W: Fundamentals of Wound Management in Surgery. Nutrition (9), 1977
10. Brooks F ed.: Gastrointestinal Pathophysiology, 2nd edn. New York; Oxford University Press, 1978
11. Elrod R: The patient with gastrointestinal disease: Disorders of the gastrointestinal tract. In: Nursing Care of the Patient with Medical-Surgical Disorders, 2nd edn., Moidel H, Giblin E, Wagner B eds. New York, McGraw-Hill, 1971, pp 726–779
12. Dunphy J: Acute abdomen. In: Current Surgical Diagnosis and Treatment, 4th edn., Dumphy J, Way L eds. Los Altos, CA, Lange Medical Publications, 1979, pp 441–449
13. Metheney N, Snively W: Perioperative fluid and electrolytes. Am J Nurs 78(2): 840–845, 1978
14. Schrock T: Small intestine. In: Current Surgical Diagnosis and Treatment, 4th edn., Dumphy J, Way L eds. Los Altos, CA, Lange Medical Publications, 1979, pp 600–625
15. Taylor V: Meeting the challenge of fistulas and draining wounds. Nursing '80, 10(1): 45–51, 1980
16. Taylor V: Gastrointestinal Diseases. Columbus, OH, Ross Laboratories, October, 1978
17. Rombeau J, Miller R: Nasoenteric Tube Feeding: Practical Aspect. Mountain View, CA, Hedeco, 1979
18. Kaminski M: Enteral hyperalimentation. J Surg Gynecol Obstet 143(1): July, 12–16, 1976
19. Dudrick S, Ruberg R: Principles and practice of parental nutrition. Gastroenterology, 61(6): 901–910, 1971
20. Ota D, Imbembo A, Zuidema G: Total parenteral nutrition. Surgery, May, 503–520, 1978
21. Borgen L: Total parenteral nutrition in adults. Am J Nurs 78(1): 224–228 1978
22. Goldstein B: Guidelines to drug incompatibilities in large volume parenterals. Nurses Drug Alert 4(8): 57–64, 1980

23. Colley R, Wilson J: Meeting patients' nutritional needs with hyperalimentation. Nursing '79, 6: 57–61, 1979
24. Sheldon G, Harper H, Way L: Surgical metabolism and nutrition. In: Current Surgical Diagnosis and Treatment, Dumphy J, Way L eds. Los Altos, CA, Lange Publishing Company, 1979, pp 160–175
25. Sorgel K, Hofmann A: Absorption. In: Pathophysiology 2nd edn., Frolich E ed. Philadelphia, JB Lippincott, 1976, pp 499–529

7 | Fluid Resuscitation of the Head-injured Patient

Diana L. Nikas

Many factors must be taken into account in the resuscitation of the head-injured patient. Two of these factors, the fluids and drugs that the patient receives, can profoundly affect intracranial dynamics, and may ultimately affect the overall outcome of the patient's condition. Fluid resuscitation cannot be addressed without taking into consideration the electrolyte status of the patient and the interplay between the pharmacologic agents given to the patient and the resultant fluid and electrolyte response.

This chapter will discuss cerebral edema in the head-injured patient, and specific, related issues which influence cerebral edema, including fluid therapy, osmotic diuretics, steroids, hypoosmolality, and hyperosmolality.

CEREBRAL EDEMA

Cerebral edema is defined as an increase in brain volume caused by an increase in water content.[1] This is differentiated from brain engorgement, which is an increase in brain volume (specifically blood volume) caused by hypoxia, hypercapnea, or venous obstruction.[1,2] However, in its advanced stages, or under conditions of impaired intracranial dynamics, cerebral engorgment can lead to vasogenic edema.[1,3]

Cerebral edema is usually classified into two categories: vasogenic or extracellular cerebral edema, and cytotoxic or intracellular cerebral edema.[1-3] Vasogenic edema is characterized by increased capillary endothelial cell permeability, causing leaking of plasma proteins and other large molecules (which are normally kept back by the blood-brain barrier) into the extracellular fluid

(ECF) space, thus enlarging the ECF volume.[1,3] Loss of autoregulation of cerebral blood flow, which occurs with breakdown of the blood-brain barrier as the result of brain injury, and arterial hypertension, both aggravate vasogenic edema.[4] In vasogenic edema, the white matter of the brain is the tissue chiefly affected, although the reasons for this vulnerability are not known.[1]

Vasogenic edema is the most common type of cerebral edema; it results from contusion, tumor, abscess, hemorrhage, infarction, and meningitis.[1,3] Vasogenic edema can cause shifting of the intracranial contents and herniation of brain tissue through a cranial defect, under the falx cerebri, over the edge of the tentorium cerebelli, or into the foramen magnum.[1,3] Clinically, the patient may demonstrate focal neurologic deficits, a depressed level of consciousness, and intracranial hypertension.

Cytotoxic cerebral edema results in intracellular swelling involving the neurons, glia, and endothelial cells, leading to a reduction of the ECF space.[1,3,4] Hypoxia produces cytotoxic edema by abolishing the ATP-dependent sodium pump within cells, causing an intracellular accumulation of sodium.[1] Water then diffuses into the cell to maintain osmotic equilibrium, resulting in intracellular volume expansion and swelling. Acute hypoosmolality caused by water intoxication, the syndrome of inappropriate ADH secretion, or acute sodium depletion also leads to intracellular swelling and cytotoxic edema.[1]

Cytotoxic edema affects both the gray and white matter of the brain; the capillary endothelial cells may also be affected, and compression of the capillary lumen may lead to increased resistance to arterial perfusion, referred to as the "no re-flow" phenomenon.[1,3]

Generalized neurologic dysfunction and increased intracranial pressure accompany cytotoxic edema. Severe cytotoxic edema caused by hypoxia may lead to cerebral infarction and associated vasogenic cerebral edema.[1]

Overgaard and Tweed[4] studied 55 head-injured patients and found that those with brain edema had significantly higher intracranial pressures than did those without edema. It was interesting to note that only 21 percent of the patients treated within 2 hours of injury developed cerebral edema, whereas 63 percent of those whose treatment was delayed for 2 to 10 hours developed edema. Delay in treatment was due to the need for transport, and these patients often presented with such untreated complications as anoxia, hypercapnea, hypotension, or mass lesions. Patients with mass lesions had a higher incidence of edema—76 percent—than did those with contusion alone—33 percent.

Overgaard and Tweed emphasized the need for adequate, early treatment of head injury and its sequelae, since ". . . this type of subacute traumatic brain edema . . . is not of major hemodynamic or clinical significance in intensively treated patients . . . ."[4] The key term here, of course, is "intensively treated patients." Overgaard and Tweed treated their patients with early surgical removal of mass lesions, controlled ventilation, and a variety of drugs reported to affect cerebral edema, including phenobarbital, furosemide, and dexamethasone. These efforts may have prevented the development of cerebral edema.

Support for this type of aggressive, early treatment comes from many sources, and its need has been illustrated in a study indicating that of 86 patients who died of avoidable causes following head injury, the most common causes of death were delayed treatment of mass lesions, uncontrolled seizures, meningitis, hypoxia, and hypotension.[5]

Besides the vitally important control of oxygenation and ventilation in the prevention of cerebral edema, it is important to determine what constitutes aggressive treatment of the head-injured patient, and those complications that are avoidable.

FLUID THERAPY

There is some controversy concerning the optimal fluid composition for resuscitation of the head-injured patient. Some authors suggest 2.5 percent glucose in 0.45 percent saline as the ideal isotonic solution for preventing cerebral edema.[2,6] Others caution against the administration of too much free water, as in the use of 5 percent dextrose in water.[2,7,8,9] It is generally agreed, however, that the patient should have restricted fluid intake. The amount of fluid recommended has varied from 800 ml/day to 1,800 ml/day, but most authors have agreed that the amount should be based on the patient's osmolality and electrolyte balance. Shenkin and co-workers[6] recommended fluid restriction to 1 liter per day of isotonic solution, maintaining that a greater fluid intake would increase the extracellular fluid space and possibly contribute to cerebral edema. They treated 10 postcraniotomy patients with an average of 1,055 ml/day of 2.5 percent glucose in 0.45 percent saline for 6 days, and found that the serum osmolality stayed within 1.5 percent of its preoperative levels, with an increase of serum sodium of only 0.8 percent. There was only a minimal increase in blood urea nitrogen (BUN) levels. Shenkin and co-workers concluded that 1 liter of isotonic fluid per day maintained patients in homeostatic fluid and electrolyte balance. No evidence of excess volume depletion occurred in these postcraniotomy patients; the authors attributed this to the inappropriate secretion of ADH (SIADH) that commonly follows craniotomy, thereby maintaining fluid balance in the face of rather severe restriction of fluid intake. SIADH has also been shown to occur following head injury, and it could thus be assumed that fluid restriction might have the same effect on these patients. Steinbok and Thompson[10] have recommended a fluid intake of 1,500 to 1,800 ml/day after finding that 5 of 6 head-injured patients who developed hyponatremia had received more than 1,800 ml/day.

Fox, Falik, and Shalhour[22] maintained their patients on 1,200 to 1,500 ml/of fluid per day using 5 percent dextrose in 0.45 percent saline. However, for patients who became hyponatremic, these authors changed to 5 percent dextrose in normal saline, since D5½NS becomes hypotonic once its dextrose content has been metabolized. This is essentially the therapy employed in our institution.

Conversely, the effects of isotonic hemodilution on cerebral edema produced by external cerebral compression in cats was examined by Jurkiewicz and Kozniewska.[34] They found that normovolemic hemodilution with Dextran 60 to a hematocrit of 25.9 ± 3.5 percent led to an increase in cerebral blood flow of 34 percent of control values. When such hemodilution was done prior to external cerebral compression, a smaller and slower decrease in cerebral microcirculation was observed. This was attributed to the decrease in blood viscosity and the decrease in peripheral resistance produced by hemodilution. The overall effect was a reduction of cerebral hypoxia (owing to improved microcirculation despite worsened oxygen content) and inhibition of the events that result in disturbance of the blood-brain barrier and cerebral edema. Whether hemodilution will be of value following head trauma to humans has not been studied.

Fluid therapy must take into account fluid losses due to injuries other than head trauma. Head-injured patients in shock should be carefully assessed for associated injuries since intracranial hemorrhage is never sufficiently extensive to produce hypovolemia in the adult.[2,11] In reviewing the causes of shock in head-injured patients, Youmans[11] found that blood loss from fractures, gunshot wounds, severe scalp lacerations or multiple trauma, hypoxia, and spinal shock was responsible for significant hypotension in 72 percent of patients. Shock due to brain injury alone was rare (3.3 percent of 654 patients) and was always accompanied by signs of brainstem involvement. Mortality rose from 10 to 90 percent when shock was produced by brain injury alone. The importance of recognizing and treating shock in head-injured patients was emphasized by the fact that hypotension was a leading extracranial cause of death in patients who had improved neurologically after injury.[5]

In addition to low blood pressure, patients with blood loss (isotonic fluid loss) will have a normal serum osmolality, sodium, and BUN, indicating isometric contraction of the intracellular fluid space. Volume replacement with blood products, and correction of the cause of fluid loss, should be done promptly.[2,5,9] Isotonic fluid volume may also be lost as third-space fluid, which results in a decrease of the ECF space and a rise in BUN, while serum sodium and osmolality remain normal. In these patients, fluid replacement with colloid solutions is necessary in order to return fluid to the vascular space and to increase the blood pressure.

Caution must be exercised against the overzealous restriction of fluids in patients who are simultaneously being treated with dehydrating agents, since this combination can lead to shock, renal failure, or both. The more obvious dehydrating agents include osmotic diuretics such as mannitol, urea, and glycerol, and loop diuretics such as furosemide and ethacrynic acid. Glucocorticoids, especially in high doses or given to glucose-intolerant patients, can also be a source of increased fluid excretion owing to the osmotic diuretic effect of high serum-glucose levels. Less obvious sources contributing to dehydration are the contrast agents used in CT (computerized tomography) scanning and angiography. These cause an osmotic diuresis and an increased urine specific gravity for 8 to 10 hours following their injection.

DIURETICS

Osmotic diuretics are often used to reduce acute increases in intracranial pressure. These agents act by creating an osmotic gradient between the cerebral vascular space and the cerebral tissues. The increase in osmolality within the vascular space pulls fluid from the interstitium of the brain into the vasculature to be excreted by the kidney. An intact blood-brain barrier is necessary for this action. Injury disrupts the blood-brain barrier; therefore normal brain tissue, rather than edematous, injured tissue, is dehydrated by these agents.[12,35] The overall effect, however, is a decrease in the total intracranial volume, and thus a decrease in the intracranial pressure (ICP).

The dosage at which osmotic diuretic agents are effective has been the source of investigation. The concern is due in part to the fact that these agents cause a sudden increase in serum osmolality and acute intravascular volume expansion when they are administered rapidly. This often causes a transient rise in ICP.[14,35]

Miller and Leech[26] used 0.5 g/kg of mannitol to demonstrate a decrease in intracranial pressure and a significant improvement in brain compliance. Levin, Duff, and Javid[16] observed that equimolar amounts of urea and mannitol (0.25 g/kg and 1.0 g/kg, respectively) were similarly effective in reducing intracranial pressure. Marshall[35] studied the effects of 0.25 g/kg, 0.5 g/kg, and 1.0 g/kg of mannitol on ICP. They found that the smaller doses (those sufficient to cause a 10 mOsm/kg rise in serum osmolality) were as effective as the larger doses in reducing ICP to normal. They and others[32] observed a transient increase in ICP with 1.0 g/kg doses of mannitol and, although no detrimental clinical effects were seen in the patients studied, this increase could have potentially disasterous effects in patients with less stable intracranial dynamics.

In addition to the effect of these agents on serum osmolality, the phenomenon of rebound has been of concern with the use of osmotic diuretics. Rebound is the increase in ICP to higher than pretreatment levels that follows dissipation of the diuretic effect of osmotic diuresis. Rebound is thought to result from the hypertonic agent entering the brain substance and creating an osmotic gradient that favors the movement of fluid from the vascular compartment into the brain tissue. In vasogenic edema that characterizes brain injury, the blood-brain barrier is impaired.[3,4,15] Since the function of the blood-brain barrier is to limit the transfer of macromolecules into the brain, its impairment may enhance the penetration of mannitol into injured tissue. There is evidence suggesting that larger doses of mannitol do have a greater potential for causing rebound,[36] although Levin, Duff, and Javid[16] reportedly observed no rebound effect with more than 500 doses of hypertonic agents administered to patients.[16]

Electrolyte changes have also been reported as complications of the use of osmotic diuretics. Both increases[17] and decreases[32] in potassium, and decreases in sodium[14] have been observed, although the levels reported remained within normal limits.

Some authors have recommended furosemide to control increased ICP, since this drug does not alter the serum osmolality, although electrolyte changes have been reported with its use.[12,17,32] The mode of action of furosemide is not clear. Its ability to decrease cerebral edema may be secondary to an associated reduced blood volume leading to diminution of hemorrhage in the lesion.[12] Experimental evidence suggests that furosemide may have a direct effect on brain tissue by suppressing active sodium transport into the edematous area,[12,17] or by decreasing the rate of CSF production,[17] or both.

The efficacy of furosemide in decreasing increased ICP has been controversial. Tornheim, McLaurin, and Sawaya[17] found decreased edema in the white matter of the contused hemisphere in experimental animals given furosemide at 3 mg/lb/day. The uninvolved hemisphere was unaffected. Cottrell and co-workers[32] recommended furosemide at 1 mg/kg and stated that it was as effective in reducing ICP as mannitol without causing changes in osmolality and electrolytes. Doses of furosemide used in experimental animals have been excessive, ranging up to 50 mg/kg, and one group of authors has admitted that this was because smaller doses had had no effect in earlier studies.[12] Other reports indicate that furosemide has been ineffective in reducing ICP, although no dose was identified and the patient population tested was extremely small.[16] Furosemide has been used in combination with other agents, including thiopental, mannitol, and steroids, in the control of ICP, with apparent success.[4,12, 6]

STEROIDS

The controversy surrounding the effectiveness of glucocorticoids in reducing the morbidity and mortality of patients with head trauma still reigns. Benson, McLaurin, and Faulkes[33] found that dexamethasone had no effect in reducing experimentally produced cerebral edema. A prospective double-blind study using placebo, low-dose (16 mg/day), and high-dose (96 mg/day) dexamethasone demonstrated no statistically significant differences in good versus bad outcome in any head-injured patients in any treatment group.[14] A regimen of high-dose methylprednisolone (two doses of 40 mg, one dose of 2 g, then 500 mg every 6 hours for 24 hours) also failed to produce improvement in head-injured patients.[18] Gobiet, and co-workers[19] also studied the effects of dexamethasone, using placebo, low-dose, and high-dose variables in head-injured patients, and found a decrease in mortality with high dose (64 to 128 mg/day) treatment. This study was critiqued by Cooper and co-workers,[14] who pointed out that the mortality differences among different groups were not statistically significant, and that the quality of survival (vegetative survival versus functional return, for example) was not analyzed. In addition, the treatment doses were given sequentially—all patients in one year received the same treatment—making observer bias and other variables a difficulty in terms of interpretation. Other studies with dexamethasone have been criticized because there were increases in the number of patients who survived in a vegetative state. In one study, when vegetative survivors were added to the mortality figures, the differences between survivors and deaths became statistically insignificant.[14]

Glucocorticoids have been shown to increase urinary output and the excretion of sodium and chloride. It is theorized that this is the mechanism responsible for the decrease in cerebral edema that is observed with use of glucocorticoids in cases of cerebral tumors.[6,18] However, since the efficacy of steroid therapy has not been established for all types of cerebral pathology, the mechanism of action of glucocorticoids has been difficult to identify.

Complications associated with glucocorticoid therapy include hyperglycemia, gastrointestinal hemorrhage, hyperosmolar coma, and an increased incidence of infection. Cooper and co-workers[14] reported a greater number of infections in patients receiving steroids, although the differences from patients not receiving steroids were not statistically significant. Others have reported a very high incidence of infection in patients receiving high-dose steroids therapy.[18] Gastrointestinal bleeding has been reported as a serious complication by a number of authors, although the incidence of this complication has varied.[13,14,18,19] Since we have been prophylactically treating patients in our neurosurgical intensive care unit with cimetidine upon their admission, we have observed a decrease in the number of patients with a heme-positive gastric aspirate and gastrointestinal bleeding. However, this is a clinical observation, and not the result of scientific study.

Reports on the incidence of hyperglycemia induced by steroid therapy have also varied, but some authors have reported glucosuria and serum glucose levels of greater than 250 mg percent, requiring temporary insulin therapy.[13,14,18,19] In my experience, hyperglycemia caused by steroids appears to be transient, is most often seen in patients receiving very high doses of glucocorticoids, and rarely requires insulin therapy. Occasionally, a patient (usually an older patient who also may be a borderline diabetic) develops glucose levels over 250 mg percent, glucosuria and, even more rarely, ketonuria, and requires insulin therapy for a short period. The importance of monitoring serum and urine glucose levels during steroid therapy is illustrated by case reports of patients who have developed hyperglycemic, hyperosmolar nonketotic coma while receiving such therapy.[20,21]

WATER AND SODIUM BALANCE

Abnormalities of sodium and water balance are the most frequently reported fluid and electrolyte changes in the neurosurgical patient,[7,10,22,23] and include the syndromes of cerebral salt wasting and cerebral salt retention. That metabolic changes should occur as the result of head injury is not surprising considering the potential for injury to the cranial structures such as the pituitary gland and hypothalamus that regulate the body's metabolic responses.[7,10]

One of the primary regulators of water balance is anti-diuretic hormone (ADH). ADH is synthesized predominantly by the supraoptic nuclei of the hypothalamus, and is stored in the posterior pituitary. The release of ADH is regulated primarily by changes in serum osmolality and circulatory volume, although many other factors also affect its release. When the serum osmolality rises, osmoreceptors in the hypothalamus are stimulated, and ADH is released from the posterior pituitary to maintain the serum osmolality at about 290 mOsm/kg. Normally, a 2 percent change in plasma osmolality is all that is necessary to produce a change from full diuresis to the initiation of antidiuresis.[24] ADH also is released when the circulating blood volume decreases or when the arterial blood pressure falls, stimulating arterial baroreceptors. When competitive forces are present, such as hypotonic hypovolemia or hypertonic hypervolemia, ADH release is modified in favor of maintaining an adequate circulatory volume and blood pressure.[24] ADH acts on the collecting ducts of the nephrons, where it causes a series of reactions leading to increased permeability of the collecting ducts and increased water reabsorption.[24]

Cerebral salt wasting (hypernatruria in the presence of hyponatremia) is more properly referred to as the syndrome of inappropriate secretion of antidiuretic hormone (SIADH), since the major defect appears to be one of water imbalance.[10] The signs of SIADH include a serum sodium osmolality of less than 275 mOsm/kg (normal: 285 to 295 mOsm/kg), a serum sodium of less than 135 mEq/L (normal: 135 to 145 mEq/L), a urine osmolality greater than the serum osmolality, and a urine sodium of more than 25 mEq/L.[7,10,22]

SIADH results from the continued secretion of ADH in the face of a decreased serum osmolality and increased circulatory volume. Since these factors normally inhibit ADH secretion, the continued release of the hormone under such circumstances is considered inappropriate. As water is reabsorbed in the kidney in SIADH, a dilutional hyponatremia occurs, producing hypoosmolality. The hypoosmolality and hyponatremia are frequently aggravated by the administration of large amounts of fluids during or after surgery.[7,22,25] Hyponatremia normally stimulates the release of aldosterone, which acts on the nephron to promote the reabsorption of sodium.

In SIADH, aldosterone secretion may be suppressed, since hypernatruria (increased excretion of sodium in the urine) also characterizes this syndrome; suppression of aldosterone secretion leads to further decrease in serum sodium and a loss of total body sodium.[7,8] This is the salt-wasting aspect of the syndrome. Expansion of the ECF volume may be the mechanism responsible for inhibiting the secretion of aldosterone and resulting in increased sodium excretion.[7,8] However, Penny and co-workers[8] have reported that investigators have suggested that hyponatremia itself acts to stimulate aldosterone release, and indeed, have found normal or elevated aldosterone levels in patients with hyponatremia. It has been hypothesized that continued loss of sodium is due to rejection of sodium at the proximal tubule (the site of most sodium reabsorption), and to an inability of the distal tubule to reabsorb all of the sodium that is presented to it, despite high aldosterone levels.[8]

Hyponatremia and hypoosmolality result in the swelling of cerebral cells owing to the osmotic gradient that is created between the extracellular and intracellular spaces, and which favors the movement of water to the area of higher concentration of solute—in this case the intracellular compartment.[7,8] Symptoms of hyponatremia may be due to the dilution of brain intracellular potassium or sodium concentrations, or both, to alterations in membrane permeability, or to cerebral edema itself.[25] The clinical signs of SIADH, therefore, are neurologic, and include loss of appetite, apathy, headache, nausea, vomiting, and irritability. In severe cases, stupor, coma, seizures, and intracranial hypertension develop.[7,8,25] Clinical signs of the syndrome are more severe with rapid changes in osmolality. Development of focal neurologic signs, especially in patients with a history of head trauma, has led to a misdiagnosis of intracranial hematoma and needless diagnostic and operative procedures.[7,8] Symptoms of hyponatremia appear to be best correlated with the interplay between net increases in brain water versus net loss of brain electrolytes.[25] Severe hyponatremia (serum Na^+ of 95 to 109 mEq/L) of 3 days duration has resulted in irreversible brain damage.[25]

Fox, Falik, and Shalhour[22] have described SIADH in 23 of 80 (29 percent) neurosurgical patients, 15 of whom had cerebral trauma. In reviewing the literature on metabolic changes in neurosurgical patients, they concluded that SIADH occurred more frequently than was recognized. Steinbok and Thompson[10] also observed SIADH in 6 of 33 severely head-injured patients.

Treatment of hyponatremia and hypoosmolality includes water restriction, and in some cases, salt administration. Steinbok and Thompson[10] recommended a fluid intake of 1,500 to 1,800 ml/day in head-injured patients in order to prevent the development of severe hyponatremia, and further fluid restriction based on the electrolyte balance of the patient. They treated patients when serum sodium levels fell below 130 mEq/L. McLaurin and King[7] also recommended fluid restriction, in addition to the administration of 20 to 40 mEq per day of sodium in an effort to prevent SIADH. Fluid restriction to 1000 ml/day was recommended for sodium levels of 115 to 125 mEq/L, and administration of hypertonic saline (6 mEq/kg of 5 percent NaCl) if neurologic symptoms developed. Arieff and co-workers[25] contended that at serum levels of less than 125 mEq/L, sublethal degrees of cerebral edema was present, even if the patient was asymptomatic. On this basis, they suggested that both fluid restriction and the administration of hypertonic saline may be appropriate; patients who were symptomatic often required both hypertonic saline and furosemide. Penny and co-workers[8] recommended fluid restriction to 800 ml/day for hyponatremia, and maintained that administration of hypertonic saline without fluid restriction would not correct the problem since the sodium would not be retained if the ECF volume remained expanded. Fox, Falik, and Shalhour[22] suggested fluid restriction alone for the treatment of SIADH if the urine sodium levels were greater than 25 mEq/L. If serum sodium was between 120 to 130 mEq/L, they restricted fluid to 600 ml/day, and changed to 5 percent saline at 6 ml/kg if neurologic symptoms developed. They added that hemodynamic monitoring would aid in adjusting fluid therapy, and that urine output and BUN should also be monitored in order to prevent excessive fluid restriction with resultant renal insult.

Hyperosmolar states have been reported to occur as often as hypoosmolar states in the neurosurgical patient.[10] Extracellular fluid tonicity determines intracellular fluid volume and since cell membranes are freely permeable to water but not to solutes, the osmolality across cell membranes is equal.[27] Therefore, hypertonic states are defined as intracellular dehydration due to increased solute concentration within the extracellular fluid space.[15,27,28] "A given cell's response to the threat of dehydration depends on the cell, the solute causing the hypertonicity and the speed with which hypertonicity develops."[27] Brain cells are unique in being able to generate new solute intracellularly, thereby drawing fluid back into themselves and returning the intracellular volume to normal. [15,27] Neither the nature of the solute formed nor its effect on cell function is known; however, experimental evidence has demonstrated that these osmoles may form in as little as 4 hours of induced cellular dehydration. [27] Nor is it known whether this is a true homeostatic mechanism or a breakdown of normal controls of intracellular solute content. [27] It must be pointed out, however, that rapid development of serum hyperosmolality may cause fatal brain dehydration before idiogenic osmoles can form.

It is not known how long it takes for the idiogenic osmoles to be removed from the brain cell when osmolality has been corrected. Rapid rehydration could produce "isotonic water intoxication" (cerebral edema) owing to cellular overhydration caused by the idiogenic osmoles pulling fluid into the cell. [27] Since intracellular fluid volume is directly related to extracellular fluid tonicity, assessment of water deficits in hypertonic states is reflected in the plasma osmolality and sodium concentration.

Hyperosmolality is caused either by water loss or solute gain, or by both. Pure water loss leads to hypernatremia and hyperosomolality in proportion to the amount of water lost. [27] This can occur as the result of inadequate water intake in patients who also have excessive water loss, such as from hyperventilation, fever, or inadequately humidified ventilators.

Central diabetes insipidus (DI) causes excessive water loss in patients who are unable to drink. Although an uncommon complication, DI may occur as the result of head trauma, especially trauma involving fractures at the base of the skull. Injury to the posterior pituitary alone causes only a transient DI, since an intact pituitary stalk is capable of releasing ADH in response to physiologic stimuli. [24] Lesions of the pituitary stalk or higher may result in degeneration of the supraoptic nuclei of the hypothalamus, leading to DI of varying severity depending on the amount of ADH that can still be released. [24] With inadequate ADH secretion, large amounts of dilute urine are excreted and, in patients who cannot replace this fluid loss, hypernatremia and hyperosmolality can develop. The diagnosis of central DI may be made on the basis of the fluid deprivation test. If, after 8 to 18 hours of fluid deprivation, the urine osmolality fails to increase above the plasma osmolality, and the plasma osmolality is greater than 300 mOsm/kg, significant ADH suppression is present. [24,29]

Central DI is treated by the administration of exogenous ADH (vasopressin). Aqueous vasopressin is a short-acting parenteral form of ADH, and is used mainly in the treatment of acute DI resulting from hypophysectomy. Vasopressin tannate in oil has a duration of 24 to 72 hours when 2.5 to 5 units are given subcutaneously, and is therefore preferred over aqueous vasopressin in the long-term control of DI. [29,30] Lysine vasopressin nasal spray is short-acting but eliminates the need for injection. It is usually ineffective in the treatment of severe DI. [29,30] DDAVP (1-deamino-8-D-arginine vasopressin) is supplied in a nasal spray and has a duration of 13 to 22 hours at doses of 10 to 20 μg; it is currently considered the drug of choice for long-term control of DI. [24,29,30] It may also be given parenterally, and does not have the pressor effects seen with

L-arginine vasopressin.[24] DDAVP may thus be the preferred drug in the acute setting, in order to avoid producing hypertension in patients with the potential for developing increased intracranial pressure.

The diagnosis of hyperosmolality due to pure water loss is based on the presence of hypernatremia, mild to moderate azotemia, a history consistent with water loss, a scant urine volume with a urine osmolality greater than that of the plasma (except in DI), and symptoms of intracellular fluid depletion.[27] Treatment is aimed at replacing water deficits, matching intercurrent water losses, and treating the cause of the water loss. Water may be replaced using D5W or D5½NS. Saline solutions that are more hypotonic than D5½NS are hemolytic and add sodium to a patient who is not sodium depleted.[27] For hyperosmolality due to pure water loss, Feig and McCurdy[27] recommended giving half of the calculated water deficit rapidly, then titrating the remainder over 1 to 2 days or longer. Neurologic deterioration after an initial improvement may indicate cerebral edema due to "isotonic water intoxication," and should this occur, treatment of water deficit should be replaced by administration of osmotic diuretics until the neurologic status has improved.[27]

Hyperosmolality can also be caused by solute gain. Solute gain is generally accompanied by water loss because the osmotic effect of extracellular solutes causes diuresis.[27] This mechanism of hypotonic fluid loss with resultant hypernatremia and hyperosmolality is commonly brought into play by high-protein tube feedings, osmotic diuretics, and hyperglycemia.[10,15,20,21,27,28,31]

Large solute loads result in acute ECF volume expansion and ICF volume contraction.[27] The osmotic diuresis thus produced leads to an isotonic urine osmolality: "Since the solute causing the diuresis constitutes a substantial fraction of the total urine solute, the electrolyte concentration of the urine must be hypotonic relative to body fluids."[27] The abrupt increase in ECF volume caused by a solute load can lead to pulmonary edema and, since the brain does not have time to generate idiogenic osmoles, cerebral dehydration occurs.[15,27]

Signs of cerebral dehydration include rather nonspecific neurologic changes: changes in the sensorium, irritability, hyperactive reflexes and, not uncommonly, seizures.[15,27] Gault and co-workers[15] reported that death was not uncommon with serum sodium levels over 185 mEq/L. Cerebral dehydration may cause mechanical stress on cerebral vessels, and may lead to such changes as small vessel thrombosis, subdural effusion, or hemorrhagic encephalopathy.[15,28] The syndrome involving hyperosmolality with hypernatremia and hyponaturia is referred to as cerebral salt retention.[15,23,28]

Authors repeatedly urge caution when administering high-protein tube feedings to patients who cannot modify their own water intake.[7,10,15,27,28] Each gram of nitrogen requires 40 to 50 ml of water for its excretion; thus dehydration occurs if inadequate water is administered with the feedings. Additionally, even a small degree of renal impairment might result in an inability of the kidney to maximally concentrate the urine, leading to an even greater water loss.[7,15] This is particularly hazardous in neurosurgical patients because such patients are usually fluid restricted, and may concomitantly be receiving osmotic diuretics, glucocorticoids, or both. Additionally, these patients frequently cannot communicate or alleviate their thirst—a major adaptive mechanism whereby the body maintains optimal osmolality. The old and the very young are particularly vulnerable to dehydration.

Among 6 hyperosmolar patients that they observed, Steinbok and Thompson[10] attributed the hyperosmolality in 1 to high-protein tube feedings. Gault and co-workers[15] reviewed the literature and found 13 cases of tube-feeding-induced hyperosmolality, 7 of whom had cerebral lesions. They also presented 3 patients under their care who had developed this problem. All 16 patients had severe hypernatrimia (as high as 192 mEq/L), moderate to marked azotemia, and a 21 to 29 percent decrease in hematocrit. Gault and co-workers[15] emphasized that serum sodium levels indicated water loss rather than a sodium excess, although an increase in total body sodium could occur as a result of the high sodium content of many tube-feeding preparations. Hyponaturia also characterized the 3 patients they presented, and may be a contributing factor in the development of hypernatremia. The mechanism leading to hyponaturia in the presence of hypernatremia may be the result of decreased extracellular volume, causing a decreased glomerular filtration rate and increased aldosterone production, although increased aldosterone levels were not a consistent finding.[15] The mechanism responsible for hyponaturia with hypernatremia may involve the natriuretic hormone of the proximal tubule, which acts independently of ADH, aldosterone, and glomerular filtration rate, and causes maximal sodium retention in these patients.[15]

The mechanism by which osmotic diuretics, such as mannitol or urea, cause hyperosmolality is essentially the same as that by which high-protein tube feedings produce the same effect. The urine excreted is hypotonic to body fluids since the greatest portion of the urine solute is mannitol or urea.[27] This results again in a greater water loss than sodium loss. Cottrell and co-workers[32] cautioned against the use of mannitol in reducing ICP because of its associated effects on osmolality and electrolytes, although the values that they reported in their study were essentially within normal limits. Marshall and co-workers demonstrated a rise in serum osmolality an average of 20 mOsm/kg with 1 g/kg doses of mannitol. McLaurin and King[7] advised monitoring serum osmolality when using osmotic diuretics, and suggested that it not be allowed to rise over 320 mOsm/kg. Prolonged osmotherapy for the treatment of cerebral edema probably is not useful since, with time, the creation of idiogenic osmoles returns the brain to its previous abnormal volumes despite continued hyperosmolality.[27] Idiogenic osmoles may also play a role, at least in part, in the rebound effect reported with mannitol and urea.

As stated earlier, hyperglycemia can occur in the head-injured patient as the result of steroid therapy.[7,14,18,19] This is especially true in older patients, patients who may be borderline diabetics, and patients in whom the stress of injury, increased cortisol levels, or exogenous steroids, proves to be more than the body can handle. These patients may require short-term insulin therapy. Gudeman, Miller, and Becker[18] reported an 85 percent incidence of hyperglycemia (serum glucose above 250 mg percent or marked glycosuria or both) in patients on high-dose methylprednisolone. Hypernatremia was seen in 15 percent of these patients and hyponatremia in 70 percent. While serum osmolalities were not reported, there is little doubt that some of these patients were hyperosmolar.

There have been case reports on hyperglycemic, hyperosmolar, nonketotic (HHNK) syndromes developing in patients receiving steroids.[20] Others have reported HHNK as a complication of cerebral compression.[21] HHNK is a syndrome of hyperglycemia (sometimes over 2,000 mg percent) leading to profound hyperosmolality, dehydration, and coma, but does not cause ketosis.[21,27] Some authors believe that ketosis does not develop because some insulin is still being produced, although in quantities inadequate to prevent hyperglycemia.[20,21]

McLaurin and King[7] found glucose intolerance in 29 head-injured patients. The possible mechanisms involved in glucose intolerance in such patients include (a) starvation; (b) increased glucose release from the liver, stimulated by cortisol; (c) decreased insulin release from the pancreas, due to suppression by catecholamines; (d) decreased peripheral utilization of glucose; (e) increased gluconeogenesis, again due to cortisol; and (f) insulin anatagonism by catecholamines.[7,20] Hyperosmolality also decreases insulin release, aggravating hyperglycemia.[27]

Increased cortisol levels have been reported in patients with head injuries and may account, in part, for rises in serum glucose levels.[7,24] The incidence, magnitude, and duration of cortisol secretion has been found to correlate positively with the severity of the head injury.[31] Exogenous dexamethasone (16 to 40 mg/day) depressed the cortisol levels in these cases, indicating that the negative feedback mechanism responsible for controlling cortisol levels was functioning, although probably not normally.[31] ACTH release stimulates cortisol secretion from the adrenal cortex, and ACTH release from the pituitary is, in turn, controlled by plasma cortisol levels—that is, by negative feedback. Since cortisol levels were abnormally high, but ACTH was still being secreted in the reported cases, it was proposed that the feedback mechanism may have been set higher. Factors that activate the pituitary-adrenal axis include: (a) hypovolemia, (b) emotions such as fear or anxiety, and (c) neural impulses from injured tissues.[31] It had been suggested that a humoral substance is released by injured tissue, and that this acts on the pituitary-adrenal axis.[31]

The expected increase in serum sodium from hypotonic fluid loss is sometimes blunted in hyperglycemia because the osmotic effect of the high glucose levels draws fluid from the intracellular to the extracellular space, causing intracellular dehydration but, at least for a time, adding fluid to the ECF space.[27] In order to assess the amount of fluid loss, the plasma sodium concentration must be corrected for the effects of the hyperglycemia—that is, it must be corrected to what the sodium concentration would be if hyperglycemia were not present[27] (see Feig and McCurdy[27] for the formulas needed for this). The corrected sodium concentration is usually elevated, indicating water loss in excess of sodium loss.[27] Although the patient with HHNK may have sodium loss in addition to water loss.[27]

Excessive hypotonic fluid loss can result in a decreased circulatory volume and hypotension. Therapy, therefore, demands immediate restoration of adequate circulatory volume, and may include plasma, blood products, or isotonic saline.[27] In addition, concurrent elimination of the causative factor— such as tube feeding or osmotic diuretic agents—is necessary. Initial resuscitation should be done rapidly to restore adequate blood pressure and urine output. In patients with normal renal function, increasing the ECF volume and blood pressure will decrease aldosterone secretion and allow urinary excretion of sodium, which will assist in the correction of hypernatremia.[27] Replacement of total volume loss and correction of hypertonicity should take place over 24 to 72 hours, in order to avoid producing isotonic water intoxication (cerebral edema).[7,15,27] Electrolyte-free water and D5½NS have been recommended.[7,27] Insulin needs in the treatment of HHNK are generally lower than those required in diabetic ketoacidosis, and insulin must be administered carefully.[21,27] Fluid therapy in HHNK may include administration of isotonic or hypotonic fluids after adequate circulatory volume has been achieved with blood or blood products.[21,27]

Finally, increased serum alcohol levels may lead to hyperosmolality, since alcohol suppresses ADH secretion and has an osmolar effect of 21.7 mOsm/L for every 100 mg percent elevation of blood alcohol.[10] Rehydration of patients with increased serum alcohol levels should be done carefully, because they may not be as dehydrated as their serum osmolality indicates. When serum osmolality values can be attained, but serum alcohol levels cannot, accurate assessment of blood alcohol levels may be calculated from the serum osmolality.[2,10]

SUMMARY

Cerebral edema is a frequent complication of head injury. Therapy aimed at preventing, diminishing, or reversing cerebral edema is controversial. Limitation of the amount of fluid intake is a generally accepted aspect of therapy, although the type of fluid to be used has not been uniformly accepted. Fluid therapy must take into account fluid loss from other causes, and should be adjusted according to serum and urine electrolytes levels and osomolality. Osmotic diuretics are known to reduce cerebral edema, although the appropriate dosage of these agents is not agreed upon. Diuretic therapy can result in fluid and electrolyte imbalances. The use of glucococorticoids in low or high doses has not consistently proven to be of benefit in head-injured patients, and the use of these drugs has resulted in hyperglycemia, gastric irritation and hemorrhage, and increased risk of infection. Cerebral salt wasting and cerebral salt retention syndromes occur with relative frequency in head-injured patients, and may be aggravated by fluid, diuretic, or steroid therapy. Sodium and water imbalances result in hypo- and hyperosmolality and changes in ECF volume; worsening of the patient's neurologic status occurs, and may compromise the potential for recovery. Careful monitoring of serum and urine sodium and osmolality may prevent these changes from having serious consequences.

REFERENCES

1. Fishman RA: Brain edema. New Engl J Med, 293:706–711, 1975
2. Roberts JR: Pathophysiology, diagnosis and treatment of head trauma. Topics Emerg Med, 1:41–62, 1979
3. Safar P: Cerebral edema. In: Critical Care Medicine Handbook, eds. Weil MH, Shubin H. New York, John H Kolen, 1974
4. Overgaard J, Tweed WA: Cerebral circulation after head injury: Part 2: The effects of traumatic brain edema. J Neurosurg, 45:292–300, 1976
5. Rose J, Valtonen S, Jennett B: Avoidable factors contributing to death after head injury. Br Med J, 2:615–618, 1977
6. Shenkin HA, Bezier HS, Bouzarth WF: Restricted fluid intake. J Neurosurg, 45:432–436, 1976
7. McLaurin RL, King LR: Metabolic effects in head injury. In: Handbook of Clinical Neurology—Injuries of the brain and skull, Part I, eds. Vinken PJ, Bruyn GW. New York, American Elvesier, 1975, pp 109–131
8. Penny MD, Walters G, Wilkins DG: Hyponatremia in patients with head injury. Intensive Care Med, 5:23–26, 1979
9. Voris HC: Craniocerebral trauma. In: Clinical Neurology, eds. Baker AB, Baker LH. Hagerstown, Md, Harper and Row, 1971
10. Steinbok P, Thompson GB: Metabolic disturbances after head injury: Abnormalities of sodium and water balance with special reference to the effects of alcohol intoxication. Neurosurgery, 3:9–15, 1978
11. Youmans JR: Causes of shock with head injury. J Trauma, 4:204–209, 1964
12. Clasen RA, Pandolfi S, Casey D: Furosemide and pentobarbital in cryogenic cerebral injury and edema. Neurology, 24:642–648, 1974
13. Marshall LF, King J, Langfitt TW: The complications of high-dose corticosteroid therapy in neurosurgical patients: A prospective study. Ann Neurol, 1:201–203, 1977
14. Cooper PR, Moody S, Clark WK, et al: Dexamethasone and severe head injury. J Neurosurg, 51:307–316, 1979
15. Gault MH, Dixon ME, Doyle M, Cohen WM: Hypernatremia, azotemia, and dehydration due to long-term high-protein tube feeding. Ann Intern Med, 68:778–789, 1968
16. Levin AB, Duff TA, Javid MJ: Treatment of increased intracranial pressure: A comparison of different hyperosmolar agents and the use of thiopental. Neurosurgery, 5:570–575, 1979
17. Tornheim PA, McLaurin RL, Sawaya R: Effect of furosemide on experimental traumatic cerebral edema. Neurosurgery, 4:48–52, 1979
18. Gudeman SK, Miller JD, Becker DP: Failure of high-dose steroid therapy to influence intracranial pressure in patients with severe head injury. J Neurosurg, 51:301–306, 1979
19. Gobiet W, Brock WJ, Liesegang J, Grate W: Treatment of acute cerebral edema with high dose dexamethasone. In: Intracranial Pressure III, eds. Beks JWF, Bosch DA, Brock M. New York, Springer-Verlag. 1976, pp 231–235
20. Boyer MH: Hyperosmolar anacidotic coma in association with glucocorticoid therapy. JAMA, 202:1007–1009, 1967
21. Davidson AR: Hyperosmolar non-ketoacidotic coma as a complication of cerebral compression. Postgrad Med J, 46:720–722, 1970
22. Fox JL, Falik JL, Shalhour RJ: Neurosurgical hyponatremia: The role of inappropriate antidiuresis. J Neurosurg, 34:506–514, 1971

23. Parent AD, Meyer GA, Tindall GT: Blood chemistry changes in head-injured patients. J Neurosurg Nurs, 4:9–20, 1972
24. Moses AM, Miller M, Streeten DHP: Pathophysiologic and pharmacologic alterations in the release and action of ADH. Metabolism, 25:697–721, 1976
25. Arieff AI, Leach, F, Massry SG: Neurological manifestations and morbidity and mortality of hyponatremia: Correlation with brain water and electrolytes. Medicine, 55:121–129, 1976
26. Miller JD, Leech P: Effects of mannitol and steroid therapy on intracranial volume-pressure relationships in patients. J Neurosurg, 42:274–281, 1975
27. Feig PU, McCurdy DK: The hypertonic state. N Engl J Med, 297:1444–1454, 1977
28. Gill W, Chapion HR, Weinstein, et al.: Serum hyperosmolality in the injured patient. Md State Med J, 27:60–63, 1978
29. Beardwell CG: The posterior pituitary and diabetes insipidus. J Clin Pathol, 7:68–71, 1976
30. Edwards CRW: Diabetes insipidus. In: Eleventh Symposium on Advanced Medicine, ed. Lant AF. London, Pittman Medical, 1975
31. Steinbok P, Thompson G: Serum cortisol abnormalities after craniocerebral trauma. Neurosurgery, 5:559–565, 1979
32. Cottrell JE, Robustelli, A, Post K, et al.: Furosemide and mannitol induced changes in intracranial pressure and serum osmolality and electrolytes. Anesthesiology, 77:28–30, 1977
33. Benson VM, McLaurin RL, Foulkes EC: Traumatic cerebral edema. Arch Neurol, 23: 179–186, 1970
34. Jurkiewicz J, Kozniewska E: Effects of hemodilution on the cerebral blood flow and blood-brain barrier in experimental cerebral oedema in cats. Resuscitation, 6:227–233, 1978
35. Marshall LF, Smith RW, Raucher LA, Shapiro HM: Mannitol dose requirements in brain-injured patients. J Neurosurg, 48:169–172, 1978
36. Stuart FP, Torres E, Fletcher R, et al.: Effects of single, repeated and massive mannitol infusions in the dog: Structural and functional changes in kidney and brain. Ann Surg, 172:190–204, 1970

SUGGESTED READINGS

Bremer AM, Yamada K, West CR: Ischemic cerebral edema in primates: Effects of acetazolamide, phenytoin, sorbitol, dexamethasone, and methyl-prednisolone on brain water and electrolytes. Neurosurgery, 6:149–154, 1980

Faupel G, Reulen HJ, Muller D, et al.: Double-blind study on the effects of steroids on severe closed head injury. In: Dynamics of Brain Edema, eds. Pappius HM, Feindel W. New York, Springer-Verlag, 1976. pp. 337–343

Kulberg G and Sundberg G: Reduction of intracranial pressure following infusion of mannitol. In: A review of clinical pressure recordings, eds. Beks JWK, Bosch DA, Brock M. Intracranial Pressure III. New York, Springer-Verlag, 1976. pp 224–227

Penn RD, Kurtz D: Cerebral edema, mass effects, and regional blood volumes in man. J Neurosurg, 46:282–289, 1977

Wise BL, Hilf R, Pileggi VJ: Fluid and electrolyte balance following injuries to the head. Am J Surg, 97:205–210, 1959

8 | Initial Hemodynamic Stabilization of the Trauma or Burn Patient

Margaret M. McMahon

An estimated 100,000 Americans die each year as a direct result of trauma; of these, 69,000 are under the age of 45. An additional 400,000 traumatized individuals suffer permanent disability.[1] The costs of trauma in terms of both physical and emotional suffering and loss to society, are incalculable. And, although substantial strides have been made in trauma care during the past decade, much remains to be done. Funding for trauma research, particularly in prevention, is pitifully small. The availability of specialized "trauma units" for the care of massively injured individuals is a fairly recent phenomenon and such units are few in number. Furthermore, unlike many medical problems, trauma is not a reportable condition, and reliable data on its incidence, treatment, and complications are thus not universally available. Finally, the provision of advanced life-support systems for the prehospital stabilization of trauma victims is confined largely to metropolitan areas.

In order for any substantial reduction in mortality and morbidity from trauma to be effected, several conditions must exist. These include rapid access of the victim to advanced life support facilities, systematic and complete assessment of the patient, implementation of a specific plan of action, and a coordinated team effort with care provided in a facility having the many resources required for both acute and long-term management.

The emphasis in this chapter is upon the initial assessment and stabilization of the patient with multiple trauma and actual or impending hypovolemic shock. The unique fluid requirements of burned individuals are also discussed.

Since prehospital advanced life support (ALS) services are not available in all communities, or are not accessed by some trauma victims even when available, it is a basic assumption in this chapter that prehospital stabilization of the trauma victim has not occurred. Furthermore, while every effort has been made to present commonly used fluid resuscitation regimens, such factors as individual physician preferences, new research, and resource availability may all influence the therapeutic approach to trauma in a given community or facility. Finally, it should be remembered that time is a major factor in the initial care of the critically injured. It is thus the norm that intervention is undertaken before assessment of the patient is complete, and thus many procedures are carried out simultaneously with assessment.

INITIAL ASSESSMENT AND RESUSCITATION

The activities of emergency personnel in the immediate postinjury phase of trauma care center upon establishing and maintaining effective airway and ventilation, restoring adequate circulatory volume and tissue oxygenation, identifying the sources and extent of blood loss, minimizing further volume loss, and providing the patient and significant others with physical and emotional preparation for surgical and other necessary procedures. Initial and repeated nursing assessment of the effectiveness of such emergency procedures is essential. Of equal importance is the recording of all assessments and interventions so that subtle changes in patient condition can be easily detected. In the multisystem injury patient, a major nursing role is coordination of the activities and orders of the many surgical specialists and other health care personnel involved and interpretation of the various care activities for the patient and significant others.

Trauma victims are special. They are physically, physiologically, and often psychologically fragile. Sudden movement or rough handling may dislodge a clot serving as the tamponaded in a major bleeding site. Failure to advise and prepare the patient before painful procedures are initiated may result in depletion of bodily resources essential to the patient's very survival. In addition to being clinically knowledgeable and technically competent, the emergency nurse must demonstrate sensitivity to the emotional needs of the patient and the patient's loved ones.

Initial Assessment

As with many other patients, the initial assessment of the trauma victim is directed at evaluating the ABCs—airway, breathing, and circulation. Life-threatening disorders affecting ventilation or circulation—such as tension pneumothorax—are remedied and obvious major bleeding is stopped. If the patient is in frank hypovolemic shock, IV fluids and oxygen are initiated. If the patient is hemodynamically stable, a rapid, 90-second, head-to-toe assessment is performed in order to detect major injuries. Since it is a normal inclination to focus on what are obvious injuries, the importance of a complete head-to-toe assessment, done systematically, cannot be overemphasized: reports of death due to major injuries which were overlooked are not uncommon.

All trauma victims with altered levels of consciousness are presumed to have cervical spine injury until proven otherwise; thus neck immobilization is accomplished first. Clothing is removed or cut away in order to adequately inspect and palpate injured areas. Unless contraindicated because of possible vertebral column injury, the patient is turned gently onto his or her side so that the back and buttocks can be examined. Failure to include this step in the initial assessment may result in failure to detect major injuries or legal evidence, including wounds of entry or exit, ecchymosis of the flank indicative of bleeding into the retroperitoneal space, surgical scars, and so forth.

Once the assessment has been completed, vital signs are taken. It should be appreciated that the initial blood pressure and pulse may be normal despite continuing blood loss. It is thus important that vital signs be measured repeatedly at 5 to 15 minute intervals. If the patient is normotensive, and it is not otherwise contraindicated, postural vital signs are taken with the patient in the supine, sitting, and possibly standing positions. While there are many disorders which may be associated with postural hypotension,[2] a decrease in the systolic blood pressure of 20 torr or more, or an increase in the pulse of 20 or more beats per minute in a trauma victim implies blood loss and the need for volume replacement.

Concurrent with or following the 90-second assessment, a history surrounding the trauma incident is obtained. In addition to obtaining of the usual patient information, including major medical problems, allergies, medications, tetanus status, and other data, details of the injury are elicited. Specific attention is directed at the mechanism of injury, since certain types of traumatic incidents are associated with well-defined injuries.[3,4,5,6,7,8,9] Vehicle speed, item of impact, use of safety belts, location in the vehicle, driver or occupant, pedestrian, and the use of alcohol or drugs are important considerations in motor vehicle accidents. In gunshot wounds, data relating to the caliber of bullet, type of weapon, distance from assailant, and position when wounded are helpful in determining the type and extent of injury. Finally, the cause of injury, if discernable, may be essential information if, for example, a motor vehicle accident was preceded by the driver experiencing chest pain. Priority might then be directed at obtaining an electrocardiogram and initiation of antiarrhythmic therapy. Finally, it is essential to know whether or not prehospital care—and especially the administration of narcotics—was provided.

Initial Intervention

The data obtained during the initial assessment determine the type and extent of intervention that follows. In the major trauma victim, efforts are directed at establishing reliable IV lines, administering of oxygen, and continuously monitoring patient during the making of decisions regarding definitive care.

Placement of IV lines   If actual or probable substantial blood loss is expected, two or more large-bore (14 or 16 gauge) around-the-needle catheters are inserted in the upper extremities of the trauma victim as far distal as possible, such as into the hands or forearms. If a more proximally placed IV catheter must be removed, and the subsequent IV site is on the arm distal to the original site, IV fluids may leak from the latter puncture site, especially when they are administered under pressure. In general, through-the-needle catheters are avoided for the same reason. Also, while radial artery cannulation is usually not performed in the initial resuscitative phase of trauma therapy, the placement of IV catheters in close proximity to the radial artery is avoided, since many major trauma victims require arterial lines later in the course of therapy.

Placement of peripheral IV lines in the trauma patient is difficult when vasoconstriction and volume depletion are present. The insertion of central venous lines via the subclavian, internal, or external jugular vein is common. Because of substantial pressure gradients, care must be taken to prevent air from entering the catheter during insertion or operation of the central venous line. "Leaving the catheter open for as short a time as two seconds in a patient making a maximal inspiratory effort can cause significant air embolus and death." [10]

In children and selected massively injured adults, IV fluids may be administered via venesection and cannulation of a femoral vein. In adults, the vein can be cannulated with standard CVP tubing. Alternatively, if the patient is essentially exsanguinated, a number 14 French nasogastric tube, or IV extension tubing with the male adaptor removed may be used for femoral vein cannulation and rapid fluid administration. In small children a pediatric feeding tube can be used under the same circumstances.

Because of the danger of thrombophlebitis and subsequent pulmonary emboli, placement of IV catheters in the lower extremities is generally contraindicated. Placement of lines in this area also creates difficulty for the anesthesiologist in reaching and monitoring such distally placed catheters. However, such distal placement is reasonable if disruption of the superior vena cava is suspected, as in the patient with massive chest trauma, for example. In children, cannulation of the saphenous vein overlying the medial malleolus is not uncommon. Whenever possible, placement of IV lines in burned or injured extremities is to be avoided. Additionally, the use of "butterfly" or scalp vein needles, although associated with a decreased incidence of thrombophlebitis, is inappropriate in resuscitation of the trauma victim. These needles are unstable, easily penetrate the vein wall causing fluid infiltration, and are not large enough to accomodate rapid fluid infusion.

An interesting but uncommon method of administering fluids in emergency situations is intraosseous administration. Valdes [11] reported the use of this method in 15 patients requiring immediate fluid administration in whom no suitable vein was available. Several of the patients receiving this treatment had conditions requiring substantial blood replacement. Both crystalloids and colloids, including whole blood, and medications were administered intraosseously. A 14-gauge needle was used for fluid administration; the sites of needle placement were the medial or lateral malleolus. No complications directly attributable to the route of fluid administration were noted.

While the major goal of treatment for the trauma victim is to quickly restore circulatory volume, it is nonetheless important that the venipuncture site be properly prepared and dressed. In addition, the use of local anesthesia prior to insertion of large-bone IV catheters is not only more humane, but also facilitates catheter insertion. Finally, when vasoconstriction or volume depletion, or both, are so pronounced that a suitable vein cannot be identified, application and inflation of the antishock suit (discussed later) may be effective is making veins accessible for cannulation.

Oxygen administration Supplemental oxygen is administered to the trauma victim via nasal prongs or a mask, at 4 to 6 liters or more per minute. Whereas use of a mask is usually desirable in order to increase the concentration of oxygen delivered, hypotensive patients often become more agitated when a face mask is in place. Modifications are made in the amount and type of oxygen delivery in patients with chronic obstructive pulmonary disease (COPD).

Foley catheter The use of a Foley catheter in the trauma victim is both diagnostic and therapeutic; it is invaluable in assessing renal function and adequacy of fluid resuscitation, and in detecting trauma involving the urinary system. Since trauma victims may have myoglobinuria or microscopic or gross hematuria, it is customary to insert a large Foley catheter, of gauge 18F or larger, in adults. Smaller catheters are easily occluded with blood clots, and maintaining their patency is difficult. A size 8 to 10 French catheter is used for children, and a straight Robinson catheter or infant feeding tube is appropriate for infants. Straight catheters must be anchored securely.

Urine output is monitored continuously and measured every 15 to 30 minutes. A urine output approximating 40 ml/hour in adults and 40 ml/m^2/hour in children is usually considered adequate. In patients with major burns or crush injuries, higher urine outputs may be desired in order to minimize renal tubular obstruction due to large myoglobin molecules.

An initial urine specimen is obtained for analysis, and repeated serial urine specimens are indicated if blood or myoglobin are present in the initial specimen. High output renal failure occurs in some patients,[12] but is usually not present in the initial resuscitative phase of therapy. Excessively high urine outputs in the absence of diuretic administration or glucosuria suggest overhydration and the need to reevaluate the rate of fluid administration. Oliguria, while occasionally due to aberrant catheter placement or blockage from blood clots, is usually interpreted as due to inadequate fluid administration.

Naso-gastric intubation As in the case of a Foley catheter, the insertion and use of a nasogastric tube is both diagnostic and therapeutic. Shunting of blood away from the splanchnic bed, as occurs in shock, may result in an adynamic ileus requiring decompression; the nasogastric tube facilitates the latter. Additionally, the drainage from a nasogastric tube is tested for blood to detect gastric trauma or preexisting conditions. In selected patients, several hundred milliliters of air may be instilled through the nasogastric tube, followed by an upright x-ray of the abdomen, for the detection of free air associated with perforation or rupture of the stomach.

Customarily, an 18 French Salem sump (double lumen) tube is used for adults. Because it has a pressure-limiting portal, the Salem sump tube can be connected to a continuous wall suction port; this obviates the need for an additional, intermittent suction apparatus.

Central venous pressure lines   Central venous pressure (CVP) lines may be inserted either for the rapid delivery of fluid, or for monitoring the adequacy of fluid resuscitation, or both. In trauma patients, CVP lines are usually centrally, rather than peripherally (as in the antecubital fossa) placed, with the subclavian or internal or external jugular veins cannulated most often.

Frequently noted causes of an abnormal CVP measurement in 'an adequately resuscitated trauma patient are aberrant catheter placement[13,14] (in the neck, pleural space, and so forth), and disorders associated with an elevated CVP, such as pericardial tamponade or tension pneumothorax. (Major complications associated with insertion or use of a CVP line are discussed in detail in Chapter 3). Administration of fluids through an aberrantly placed catheter in the chest may cause hydrothorax or hydromediastinum[15] and pronounced respiratory embarassment, in addition to inadequate fluid resuscitation. The complications associated with centrally placed CVP lines are summarized in Table 8-1.

The range of normal CVP is 5 to 12 cm H_2O, with the reading taken at end-expiration, the base of the manometer placed at the correct zero point, and with the patient in the supine position. Knopp and Dailey recommend a zero point as located at ''40–45% of the anterior-posterior diameter of the chest, measured anterior to posterior at the fourth intercostal space to approximate the location of the tricuspid valve.''[15] The zero point selected is marked on the patient's chest so that subsequent CVP measurements will be obtained from the same location.

It is important to appreciate that changes in the CVP are of more value than is a single CVP reading in determining the adequacy of volume resuscitation. In the initial stages of resuscitation, CVP measurements are obtained every 5 minutes or more frequently, as needed. If frequent measurements are needed, it is essential that an additional IV line be placed, since each CVP measurement disrupts fluid resuscitation efforts.

As soon as possible after CVP catheter insertion, a chest x-ray is obtained to verify the correct placement of the catheter. All catheter and manometer connections must be well secured with adhesive tape to prevent inadvertent disruption of the system and subsequent air embolus.

Recording   In order for the data obtained from both invasive and noninvasive monitoring to be of value in analyzing the response of the trauma patient to therapy, assessments and interventions must be recorded in a clear, concise, and accessible manner. A variety of trauma ''flow sheets'' have been designed for this purpose and are invaluable in communicating essential information to other treatment team members. Some agencies also utilize a large, white board, visible to all in the treatment room, to communicate information about the patient. Information recorded on the board may include the most recent vital signs, lab

TABLE 8-1. Complications Associated with
Centrally Placed (Subclavian and Internal
Jugular) Central Venous Pressure Catheters

Pneumothorax
Arterial puncture
Bleeding from catheter site
Air embolus
Brachial plexus injury
Internal mammary injury[a]
Thoracic duct injury
Osteomyelitis of clavicle[a]
Phrenic injury
Vagus injury
Horner's syndrome

[a]Subclavian cannulation only.
From Knopp R, Dailey RH: Central venous can-
nulation and pressure monitoring. Journal of the
American College of Emergency Physicians, re-
cently changed to Annals of Emergency
Medicine, 6:358–366, 1977.

values, amount of blood ordered, and fluids administered. Such a communication system serves to decrease confusion and to minimize the noise level in both
the treatment room and the emergency department.

OTHER STABILIZATION MEASURES

Once the immediate goals of resuscitation and stabilization of the trauma
patient have been achieved, attention is directed to minimizing further blood loss
and complications by providing for immobilization of fracture sites and performing wound care. Long-bone fractures are associated with an increased
incidence of fat emboli,[16,17] laceration or spasm of major vessels, and nerve
damage. In addition, fracture immobilization is helpful in decreasing or
eliminating pain in the affected area.

Injury with or without fracture may result in substantial tissue swelling and
impairment of vessel patency and nerve function. Such swelling is of particular
concern when it occurs within fascial compartments, with the term "compartmental syndrome" used to describe the disorder. Compartmental syndrome
is characterized by extreme tenseness of the tissues in the injured area, pain with
active and passive movement of such distal structures as the fingers or toes, pain
that is severe and out of proportion to the injury, and often, but not always,
decreased circulation and capillary refill of the distal extremity. While this
syndrome may result from trauma to any of the fascial compartments, those of
the forearm and lower leg are particularly vulnerable.[17] Prevention of compartmental syndrome includes prompt immobilization, splinting, and elevation
of the injured extremity, and the application of ice to minimize swelling. Once
compartmental syndrome has occurred, the extremity is placed level with the
heart (since continued elevation will further impede blood supply), and surgical

decompression by fasciotomy is done promptly. It is imperative that the distal pulses in injured extremities be marked with an "X" and palpated frequently.

Wound care of the burned individual varies from institution to institution. At the very least, personnel working in proximity to such patients should wear surgical gowns, masks, and gloves, and use sterile technique when providing care. Once adequacy of the airway and ventilation have been established, attention is directed at removing items which retain heat, such as clothing, jewelry, and the like. If possible, the treatment room should be heated or a heat shield should be used. Prevention of hypothermia is an important consideration during resuscitation of the burn victim and burn wound care, especially in infants and small children.

Burned areas may be gently cleansed with a dilute concentration of povidone-iodine without detergent (that is, prep solution, not scrub solution) followed by irrigation with an isotonic solution such as normal saline or Tissusol. Debridement of loose tissue and application of a topical agent, such as silver sulfadiazene, may or may not be done initially, depending on whether or not transfer of the patient to a burn unit is anticipated, and depending also upon the time delays involved in any transfer. In burned individuals requiring immediate surgery, the wound care is usually accomplished in the operating room. Unless there has been or will be a substantial delay in the time from injury to burn wound treatment in a burn unit, application of topical agents is usually not warranted in the emergency room. Regardless of whether or not dressings have been applied, the burn patient should be covered with clean sheets followed by clean blankets to conserve body heat.

Wounds other than burns are cleansed and irrigated with an isotonic solution and dressed. In general, the definitive care of wounds is accomplished only after all diagnostic studies have been completed and the patient is clearly hemodynamically stable. As with the burn victim, lacerations in persons requiring immediate surgery are repaired in the operating room. It is important that the surgery personnel be alerted to the extent of such surface trauma and to the requirements for operative care.

It is interesting to note that studies of the quality of major trauma care, particularly in rural areas, have indicated that wound care and fracture immobilization are given a higher priority than is appropriate, often superseding the care of other, more life-threatening injuries.[18,19,20] Cosmesis is relegated to a very low priority in the management of the major trauma victim.

DIAGNOSTIC STUDIES

Since the availability of whole blood for rapid infusion may be a major factor in the survival of the trauma patient, priority is given to obtaining blood specimens for typing and crossmatching. Usually the blood is drawn when the first IV is inserted. While the number of units required varies, 4 to 10 units are requested in massively injured adults. In communities with prehospital advanced life support facilities, blood specimens for type and crossmatch may be drawn at the scene and rapidly transported by police or other official vehicle to the hospital or blood bank. When this system is used it is not uncommon for the typed and crossmatched blood to arrive before or shortly after the patient reaches the emergency department.

Other laboratory studies obtained on the trauma patient include the CBC, electrolytes, BUN, glucose, coagulation screen, amylase, urinalysis, arterial blood gases, and a 12-lead electrocardiogram (ECG). An ECG and cardiac monitoring are important in the assessment and management of all major trauma victims, and particularly those with blunt trauma to the chest. It is helpful to appreciate that ECG evidence of myocardial damage has been noted in the absence of external signs of chest trauma.[21,21]

In patients with unexplained altered levels of consciousness, evidence of drug or alcohol intake, or a history suggesting drug or alcohol abuse, blood alcohol or other toxicology studies are indicated. Carboxyhemoglobin levels are measured in selected burn victims. When intraabdominal bleeding is suspected and a peritoneal lavage is performed, the aspirated fluid is analyzed for RBCs, WBCs, amylase, and bacteria. Recent research by Oppenheim, and co-workers[21] suggests that blood lactate, pyruvate, and alanine values may be helpful is assessing severity of injury during the early hours of trauma, and may be useful indicators in determining deterioration in the patient's condition. The extent to which these studies are currently employed is unclear, but their value in trauma care appears to warrant consideration.

Because time is crucial in treatment of the trauma victim, and priorities may have to be established for laboratory personnel, laboratory request slips may be stamped with a large and clearly visible alert or caution statement, such as "major trauma, priority #1." In a similar mode, some hospitals cover all trauma victims and seriously ill medical patients with a red blanket; priority for x-ray and use of the elevator then become quite evident to both personnel and visitors.

Radiographic studies required in the assessment of the trauma victim vary, but the taking of at least chest and abdominal films is routine. Whenever cervical-spine injury is suspected, a cross-table lateral film of the neck, with the patient kept on the stretcher, is taken and read first. Once the cervical-spine is "cleared," other films may be taken. It should be emphasized that the role of x-ray personnel in trauma cases is to take x-rays, not to take care of the patient. Trauma victims must be stabilized prior to leaving the emergency department, and must have continuous nursing assessment while having x-rays. In a review of deaths following abdominal trauma due to motor vehicle accidents, Foley and co-workers[3] noted two consistent factors: (a) a failure to adequately volume-resuscitate the patients and to appreciate continued blood loss; and (b) the death of many patients while in the x-ray department. Clearly the risk-benefit factors in taking x-rays must be evaluated in seriously injured individuals, and thought must be given to the efficacy of doing radiographic studies directly in the operating room.

VOLUME RESUSCITATION

Despite the travesty of the Vietnam conflict, lessons learned in the management of massively injured individuals have been transferred to the civilian community and have resulted in the saving of many lives. The principles of rapid access and transport, and of field stabilization have effected a substantial increase in the number of massively injured persons who, in the past, would have expired, arriving alive at hospital emergency departments. This and improved surgical techniques and technology have created new challenges in trauma therapy, and a myriad of complications rarely seen 10 years ago. One of the most signficant and perplexing of the latter is the adult respiratory distress syndrome (ARDS).

Much attention has been given to, and research generated in, the prevention and treatment of ARDS; a variety of etiologies and fluid resuscitation protocols have been proposed. Discussed briefly in this section are some of the fluid resuscitation guidelines currently in use. It is important to appreciate that controversy in the treatment of ARDS abounds, and that research on the syndrome is ongoing; treatment regimens may change quickly. Thus it behooves the reader to seek current information in this regard.

Ringer's Lactate

Research by Shires and co-workers,[12,24] Pirkle,[25] and many others suggests that patients experiencing large blood loss have both intravascular and interstitial volume loss, with some of the interstitial fluid being shifted to the cells, as depicted in Figure 8-1. Accordingly, replacement of lost blood with whole blood alone produced inadequate resuscitation. The addition of a balanced salt solution containing electrolytes improved the survival of animals subjected to shock/blood loss studies (Fig. 8-2).

Because of factors such as the foregoing, it is common that the initial fluid selected for volume replacement in trauma cases is Ringer's lactate. In the hypotensive trauma patient, 1 to 2 liters of this are infused rapidly, usually over a 30 to 40 minute period. A systolic blood pressure of 90 to 100 torr is desired. If no response is noted, an additional fluid challenge is made. A failure to respond, or continued deterioration of the patient may suggest concomitant or isolated cardiogenic shock. If the vital signs improve and then deteriorate, there may be a strong likelihood that the blood loss is continuing and can only be contained surgically. It should be appreciated that the replacement of lost blood by crystalloid does not follow a one-to-one relationship. A loss of 1 liter of blood may require 3 to 5 liters of Ringer's lactate for adequate resuscitation of the patient. Recent research by Peters and Hogan[26] suggests that while the total volume of crystalloid administered may be a factor in the development of ARDS, the *rate of fluid administration* may be the more critical factor in the development of high-permeability pulmonary edema.

NORMAL

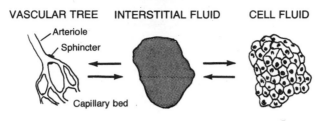

HEMORRHAGIC SHOCK

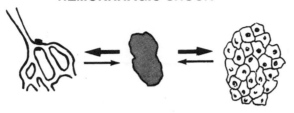

Fig. 8-1.   Conceptual illustration of interstitial fluid response to hemmorrhagic shock (From: Shires GT, Carrico CJ, Canizaro PC: Shock. Vol. 13, Major Problems in Clinical Surgery. Philadelphia, WB Saunders, 1973.)

Normal Saline

Normal saline is used for the initial resuscitation of the trauma victim, and is administered in much the same way as Ringer's lactate solution. The use of saline rather than Ringer's lactate appears to be based more on individual physician preference that on any research-substantiated superiority of saline over Ringer's lactate. Its use, however, may be indicated in selected patients with electrolyte excesses.

Five Percent Dextrose in Ringer's Lactate

Ringer's lactate containing dextrose is commonly used in individuals who do not have substantial blood loss, and in some institutions, in multiple trauma patients who also have head injury.

Whole Blood

Once fluid resuscitation has been initiated with Ringer's lactate and there is evidence of a continuing need for volume replacement, whole blood is added to the fluid regimen. While type-specific, crossmatched blood is the most desirable blood for this purpose, type-specific uncrossmatched blood may be used in urgent situations. Alternatively, O-negative blood may be used. In some instances, such as military combat, disaster situations, and others, O-positive,

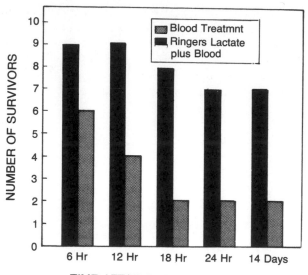

Fig. 8-2.   Comparison of effects of blood replacement alone with Ringer's lactate plus blood on the survival of dogs with hemorrhagic shock (From: Shires GT, Carroco CJ, Canizaro PC: Shock. Vol. 13, Major Problems in Clinical Surgery. Philadelphia, WB Saunders, 1973.)

low-antibody-titer blood may be infused. O-positive, low-titer blood was used extensively during the Vietnam conflict without apparent serious complication.

Since it is theorized that the infusion of multiple thrombi and debris from banked blood may be a factor in the development of ARDS, attention has been directed at the inclusion of various specialized filters in transfusion tubing.[27] Also suggested have been frequent changing of the standard initial blood filter. Stith[28] recommends changing the filter and tubing for every 3 to 4 units of blood administered or more frequently if the flow is impeded. The relative benefits of specialized in-line ultrafilters compared with the delays in infusion time and the patient cost are factors that must be considered. The inclusion of ultrafilters may result in a decrease in the rapidity with which blood can be administered[27]; and those filters that are most effective in filtering out debris may also slow the flow rate to the greatest extent.[27] Decisions must therefore sometimes be made on a case-by-case basis in regard to the importance of minimizing microaggregates as compared with the urgency of whole blood replacement.

Albumin

Albumin is used in several different ways in the management of trauma victims. It may be administered when whole blood is totally unavailable, or when there is a time delay before the arrival of whole blood and the patient cannot be sustained with Ringer's lactate. A fairly new use of albumin is that proposed by Jelenko and co-workers[29] known as the HALFD method of volume repletion.

HALFD is an acronym for the hypertonic albuminated fluid demand regimen for burned or traumatized individuals. The solution used and the guidelines for determining the rate of fluid administration are listed in Figure 8-3. The conclusions of Jelenko and co-workers, based on a study of 38 burned patients, were that: "patients treated with the HALFD method fared significantly better clinically, needed less fluid, had less weight gain and plasma leak, and experienced slower volume repletion than those treated more traditionally. We conclude that the HALFD method is a physically and physiologically appropriate paradigm for resuscitating the volume-depleted patient."

Dextran

The use of both low- and high-molecular-weight dextran in the management of trauma victims is largely confined to situations in which whole blood is unavailable. The duration of effectiveness of dextran in expanding the circulatory volume rarely exceeds 48 hours.[12] Major concerns with dextran are that it may interfere with clotting, thus contributing to or potentiating serious bleeding diatheses, and may precipitate allergic reactions including anaphylaxis. If dextran must be used, it is imperative that adequate blood be obtained for type and crossmatch before the dextran is administered; the anticlotting properties of dextran may interfere with the type and crossmatch procedure.

Artificial Blood: Fluosol-DA

The major shortcoming of non-blood plasma expanders has been their inability to transport oxygen. It appears that this obstacle has been overcome with the introduction of Fluosol-DA. This substance is a perfluorochemical with oxygen-carrying capabilities, and has been used successfully in a limited number of patients in Japan and the United States. At present, the use of this product requires authorization of the Food and Drug Administration, and its distribution is limited. Studies with Fluosol-DA involving healthy volunteers[30] and severely anemic patients[31,32,33] have failed to discern complications or toxicity. The role of Fluosol-DA in the management of trauma is speculative at best, but it seems most likely that it will be limited to situations in which blood is unavailable or is refused by patients on the basis of religious beliefs, as in the case of Jehovah's Witnesses.

ADJUNCTS IN THE RESUSCITATION OF TRAUMA VICTIMS

Anti-shock Suit

The anti-shock suit, known also as MAST trousers (military anti-shock trousers) or a G-suit, is a device gaining considerable popularity in the immediate resuscitation of the victim of hypovolemic shock. The device is a three-

The Fluid (HALFD)

To 1000 ml 5% D/W or sterile water for injection add:
120 mEq NaCl
120 mEq Na lactate
12.5 g (50 ml) serum albumin (Ab)

The Method

A. Infuse the fluid so that:

1. $MAP = \left[\dfrac{(BP_s - BP_d)}{3}\right] + BP_d \geqslant 60 \leqslant 110$ torr—preferably $\pm$ 70–75 torr

2. Urine volume (UV) $\geqslant 30 \leqslant 50$ ml/hr based on q 15 min collections.
3. Pulse pressure 40 torr

B. Follow the laboratory results:

1. Serum Na^+ and K^+ q 4H.
2. When $Na^+ \geqslant 148$ mEq/dl $\leqslant 152$ mEq/dl switch to 0.25 N NaCl + 12.5 gm Ab. still keeping $\overline{MAP}$ and UV in same range as A2.
3. If K^+ drops 0.3 mEq/dl, add KCl to infusate in 20-40 mEq/l increments.
4. When patient can maintain fluid needs by mouth, stop IV fluid.

Fig. 8-3.   Noninvasive determination of the rate of fluid administration using the hypertonic albuminated fluid demand (HALFD) method (From: Jelenko C, et al.: Shock and Resuscitation II: Volume repletion with minimal edema using the "HALFD" method. J Am Coll Emerg Phys 7:326–333 1978.)

compartment pneumatic suit which is applied to the legs and abdomen (Fig. 8-4) of the victim. When the suit is inflated, blood from the legs and abdomen is shunted into the more vital areas of the body, and the blood pressure, pulse, and perfusion are improved. In an adult, inflation of all three compartments of the suit may result in a blood pressure rise equivalent to a 750 to 1000 ml increase in the blood volume.[34] Hazards associated with the suit are few, and complications more often relate to a lack of knowledge in its use on the part of in-hospital professional personnel than from errors in the pre-hospital phase of care.

Improvements in blood pressure and perfusion as a result of use of the anti-shock suit are temporary; precipitous deflation of the suit, without appropriate volume replacement, will return the patient to a hypotensive state. The suit is therefore deflated gradually, with IV fluids concurrently administered to return or maintain the blood pressure at the pre-deflation level. X-rays may be taken with the suit in place; the design of the suit allows access to the perineal area for urinary bladder catheterization.

In addition to improving blood pressure and perfusion, the anti-shock suit is also useful for tamponading major bleeding of the abdomen, legs, or both, and for immobilizing fractures of the pelvis. It may be of limited value in immobilizing fractures of the femoral shaft.

The applicability of the anti-shock suit in differentiating hypovolemic shock from cardiogenic shock has been reported by Wayne.[35] Whereas an estimated 20 to 30 percent of patients with cardiogenic shock also have hypovolemic shock, the use of the MAST suit serves as a reversible fluid challenge. The efficacy of the MAST suit in decreasing the mortality associated with cardiogenic shock remains to be determined.

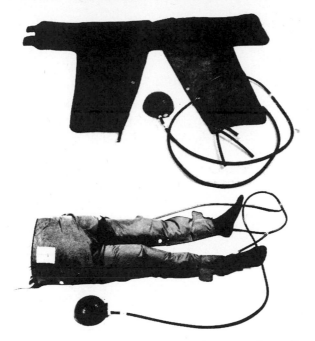

Fig. 8-4.   (Top) MAST trousers in position for receipt of patient. (Bottom) Trousers inflated on patient (From: McSwain NE: Pneumatic trousers and the management of shock. J Trauma 17:719–724, 1977.)

Contraindications to use of the anti-shock suit are relative. In general, persons with congestive heart failure or substantial head or chest trauma are not candidates for the suit, nor are pregnant women. If the patient has no palpable blood pressure, however, brain perfusion can only be improved through the effects of the suit. In pregnant women or persons with grossly obese abdomens, the abdominal compartment can be left uninflated. Finally, the anti-shock suit is expensive; care must be taken to prevent damage to the bladders by glass, scissors, needles, or scalpels.

Autotransfusion

Autotransfusion is the recovery, filtration, and return to the patient, by infusion, of the patient's own shed blood. Blood shed into the pleural space following blunt or penetrating chest trauma is most commonly transfused; however, the recent experience of Glover and colleagues[36] suggests that the autotransfusion of blood contaminated by intestinal contents may also be lifesaving in specific instances.

Depending upon the system used, such as in the case of a continuous circuit with the body, as opposed to reservoir collection, autotransfusion may be acceptable to Jehovah's Witnesses. A discussion of the nursing and equipment requirements associated with autotransfusion is beyond the scope of this chapter, and the reader is urged to review the work of Hollingsworth[37] for specific information.

Intracranial Pressure Monitoring

Fluid resuscitation of the trauma victim experiencing concomitant head injury is difficult at best. In order to minimize cerebral edema, a fine balance must be maintained between adequate volume replacement and fluid restriction. Changes in the level of consciousness and vital signs, which are indicative of increasing intracranial pressure, occur late and are masked or obliterated by shock and anesthesia. Intracranial pressure monitoring following the resuscitation of patients has indicated in many instances that the intracranial pressure was already well above acceptable limits,[38] thus suggesting that there was the need to initiate such monitoring earlier in order to effect a change in mortality and morbidity. The insertion of subarachnoid screws for intracranial pressure monitoring is gaining in popularity as an integral part of the emergency department resuscitation of the head-injured patient. At this time, however, the majority of intracranial pressure monitoring occurs in the intensive care unit.

FLUID RESUSCITATION OF THE BURN VICTIM

Although many of the therapeutic principles and interventions previously discussed in this chapter have relevence for the burn victim, special attention must be directed at the unique fluid needs of these patients. A variety of fluid resuscitation regimens have been proposed in the initial management of the patient with major burns, and controversy continues over the most effective protocols. The use of the HALFD method employed by Jelenko and colleagues was discussed earlier. Some interest has also been generated in the use of hypertonic saline solutions, although their acceptance is not widespread.

The most commonly used formula for fluid replacement in the immediate care of the individual with major burns, covering greater than 20 percent of the body surface area (BSA), is Ringer's lactate administered at a rate adequate to deliver 4 ml/kg/percent BSA burned within the first 24 hours. One half of the 24 hour requirement is administered within the first 8 hours after the burn is sustained. The second half of the fluid requirement is delivered over the next 16 hours. It is essential to remember that the volume delivered in the first 8 hours is marked from the time of the burn injury, and not from the time that the patient is first seen in the emergency care setting. A failure to accommodate for time delays may result in substantially inadequate volume replacement. The fluid requirement for the second 24 hours is normally one half of the requirement of the first 24 hours. Colloid, in the form of albumin, is usually not administered in the first 12 to 24 hours. Likewise, whole blood also is not administered unless the patient has experienced other trauma causing blood loss. While burn-induced hemolysis does occur, it is most often a late rather than an immediate concern.

The fluid requirements of children, and of persons experiencing electrical burns may differ from those listed above. Consultation with burn specialists is indicated early in the care of these individuals. As with the trauma victim, the actual parameters used to assess the adequacy of volume replacement in the electrical burn victim are the sensorium, urine output, normal body temperature, and a normal CVP. Assessment of the patient is the key because fluid requirements often exceed those calculated initially.

PAIN MANAGEMENT IN THE TRAUMA OR BURN VICTIM

Providing for pain relief in the massively injured or burned individual is an understandable concern. However, what personnel interpret as pain in the trauma victim may actually be hypoxia-induced agitation or confusion. The effects of narcotics or other analgesics may precipitate or compound hypovolemia, and these substances are best avoided until the patient is adequately fluid-resuscitated. In both massive trauma and burn patients, narcotics are administered intravenously in small doses, with careful monitoring of vital signs. The anesthesiologist should be consulted in decisions about narcotic administration when surgery is anticipated.

Nonnarcotic creative approaches to pain relief warrant consideration. The self-administered inhalation of a combination of nitrous oxide and oxygen (Dolonox) has been effective in relieving pain in a variety of etiologies including myocardial infarction and major burns, without producing serious effects on vital signs. Therapeutic touch has been employed in the relief of pain due to musculoskeletal trauma, and its value in major trauma and burn patients warrants attention.[39] Providing the patient with information and reassurance, and allowing significant others to remain with the patient, may be equally as or more effective than the use of narcotics.

PREVENTION

While the primary goal of emergency-care is the resuscitation of the critically burned or injured, one should seize every opportunity to provide education of the patient and significant others in the prevention of trauma. How many more helmetless motorcyclists will die or live vegetatively before the message of head injury is received, understood, and accepted? Nor are seat belts a nuisance; they are a necessity.

In addition to patient education in the prevention of trauma, professionals are encouraged to support, and be involved in, the activities of such organizations dedicated to the prevention of trauma as the American Trauma Society and countless others. The incredible loss of life or function that occurs each year as the result of trauma cannot be reduced without the commitment and involvement of health care providers and consumers alike.

REFERENCES

1. Cowley RA: Why not a national institute for trauma? (Third Annual Stone Lecture, American Trauma Society). J Trauma, 19:354–357, 1979
2. Bookman LB, Simoneau JK: The early assessment of hypovolemia: postural vital signs. J Emerg Nurs, 3:43–46, 1977
3. Foley RW, Harris LS, Pilcher DL: Abdominal injury in automobile accidents: review of care of fatally injured patients. J Trauma, 17:611–615, 1977
4. Frey C: Initial Management of the Trauma Patient. Philadelphia, Lea and Febiger, 1976
5. Gratz RR: Accidental injury in childhood: a literature review on pediatric trauma. J Trauma, 19:551–555, 1979
6. Greenberg MI: Falls from heights. J Am Coll Emerg Phys, 7:300–301, 1978
7. Lenoski EF, Hunter KA: Specific patterns of inflicted burn injuries. J Trauma, 17:841–846, 1977
8. Weis EB, Printz HB, Hassler CR: Experimental automobile-pedestrian injuries. J Trauma, 17:823–828, 1977
9. Zettas JP, et al.: Injury patterns in motorcycle accidents. J Trauma, 19:833–836, 1979
10. Walt AJ, Wilson RF: Management of Trauma: Pitfalls and Practices. Philadelphia, Lea and Febiger, 1975
11. Valdes MM: Intraosseous fluid administration in emergencies. Lancet, 2:1235–36, 1977
12. Shires GT, Carrico CJ, Canizaro PC: Shock, Vol. 13, Major Problems in Clinical Surgery. Philadelphia, WB Saunders, 1973
13. Arbitman M, Kart BH: Hydromediastinum after aberrant central venous catheter placement. Crit Care Med, 7:27–29, 1979
14. Krausz MM, et al.: Aberrant position of a central venous catheter: A cause for inadequate fluid replacement in septic shock. Crit Care Med, 6:337–338, 1978
15. Knopp R, Dailey RH: Central venous cannulation and pressure monitoring. J Am Coll Emerg Phys, 6:358–366, 1977
16. Lahiri B, Wallock RZ: The early diagnosis and treatment of fat embolism syndrome. J Trauma, 17:956–959, 1977
17. Nixon RJ, Brock-Utne JG: Free fatty acid and arterial oxygen changes following major injury. J Trauma, 18:23–26, 1978
18. Houtchens BA: Major trauma in the rural mountain west. J Am Coll Emerg Phys, 6:343–346, 1977
19. Houtchens BA: Initial evaluation and management of major trauma in the rural setting: An appeal for a "national standard." J Leg Med, 5:38–44, 1977
20. Moylan JA, et al.: Evaluation of the quality of hospital care for major trauma. J Trauma, 16:517–523, 1976
21. Miller MS, Scott FC: Cardiac contusion and right bundle branch block. J Am Coll Emerg Phys, 6:504–506, 1977
22. Weisz GM, et al.: Electrocardiographic changes in traumatized patients. J Am Coll Emerg Phys, 5:329–331, 1976

23. Oppenheim WL, et al.: Early biochemical changes and severity of injury in man. J Trauma, 20:135–140, 1980
24. Shires GT: Management of hypovolemic shock. Bull NY Acad Med, 55:139–149, 1979
25. Pirkle JC, Gann DS: Expansion of interstitial volume is required for full restitution of blood volume after hemorrhage. J Trauma, 16:937–947, 1976
26. Peters RM, Hogan JS: Mechanism of death in massive fluid infusion. J Trauma, 20:452–459, 1980
27. Rosario MD, et al.: Blood microaggregates and ultrafilters. J Trauma, 18:498–506, 1978
28. Stith H: Personal communication. Seattle, Washington, July, 1980
29. Jelenko C, et al.: Shock and resuscitation II: volume repletion with minimal edema using the "HALFD" method. J Am Coll Emerg Phys, 7:326–333, 1978
30. Ohyanagi H, et al.: Clinical studies of perflourochemical whole blood substitutes: Safety of Fluosol-DA (20%) in normal volunteers. Clin Ther, 2:306–312, 1979
31. Gonzalez ER: Fluosol a special boon to Jehovah's Witnesses. JAMA, 243:720, 724, 1980
32. Gonzalez ER: The saga of "artificial blood." JAMA, 243:719–720, 1980
33. Maugh TH: Blood substitute passes its first test. Science, 206:205, 1979
34. McSwain NE: Pneumatic trousers and the management of shock. J Trauma, 17:719–724, 1977
35. Wayne MA: The MAST suit in the treatment of cardiogenic shock. J Am Coll Emerg Phys, 7:107–109, 1978
36. Glover JL, et al.: Autotransfusion of blood contaminated by intestinal contents. J Am Coll Emerg Phys, 7:142–144, 1978
37. Hollingsworth P: Autotransfusion in the emergency department. J Emerg Nurs, 3:9–12, July/Aug 1977
38. Palmer MA, et al.: Intracranial pressure monitoring in acute neurologic assessment of multi-injured patients. J Trauma, 19:497–501, 1979
39. Sandroff R: A skeptic's guide to therapeutic touch. RN, 43:24–83, 1980

SUGGESTED READINGS

American College of Surgeons Committee on Trauma: A guide to the initial therapy of shock. Consultant, 18:94, 1978

Ballinger WF II, Rutherford RB, Zuidema GD (eds.): The Management of Trauma, Philadelphia, WB Saunders, 1973

Barry J: Emergency Nursing. New York, McGraw-Hill, 1978

Berg BC, Danzl DF: Peritoneal lavage and scintigraphic evaluation of blunt abdominal trauma. J Am Coll Emerg Phys, 6:397–404, 1977

Cameron CTM: Nonresuscitative aspects of the management of severe injuries. JACEP, 7:313–314, 1978

Champion RH, Sacco WJ, Lepper RL, et al.: An anatomic index of severity. J Trauma, 20:197–202, 1980

Ciancutti AR: Emergency Care Handbook. Westport, Connecticut, Technomic Publishing, 1977

Detmar DE, Moylan JA, Rose J, et al.: Regional categorization and quality of care in major trauma. J Trauma, 17:592–599, 1977

Dillman PA: The biophysical response to shock trousers. J Emerg Nurs, 3:21–23, 1977

Drury LR: Evacuation and early care of the trauma patient. Heart and Lung, 7:249–252, 1978

Gay P, Thede J, Suehiro G, McNamara JJ: Filtration of debris from banked blood. J Trauma, 19:806–811, 1979

Hathaway R: Hemodynamic monitoring in shock. J Emerg Nurs, 3;37–40, 1977

Haughey B: CVP lines: Monitoring and maintaining. Am J Nurs, 78:635–638, 1978

Jay KM, Bartlett RH, Danet R, Allyn PA: Burn epidemiology: a basis for prevention. J Trauma, 17:943–947, 1977

Jones CA: Emergent care of burn victims. J Emerg Nurs, 1;13–16, 1975

Kaplan BC, Civetta JM, Nagel EL, et al.: The military anti-shock trouser in civilian pre-hospital emergency care. J Trauma, 13:843–847, 1973

Katsaros C, Bobb J: Shock—The critical hour. J Emerg Nurs, 4:45–50, 1978

Lindsey D: Teaching the initial management of major multiple system trauma. J Trauma, 20:160–162, 1980

Markovchick VJ, Evans GT, Rosen P, et al.: Traumatic acute pericardial tamponade. J Am Coll Emerg Phys, 6:562–567, 1977

McFarland MB: Fat embolism syndrome. Am J Nurs, 76:1942–1944, 1976

McKnight W: Understanding the patient in emergency. Can Nurs, 72:20–23, 1976

McMahon MM: Physiologic shock. In: Medical-Surgical Nursing: A Psychophysiologic Approach, 2d edn., eds. Luckmann J, Sorensen KC. Philadelphia, WB Saunders, 1980

McMahon MM: Medical-surgical emergency nursing. In: Medical-Surgical Nursing: A Psychophysiologic Approach, 2d edn., eds. Luckmann J, Sorensen KC. Philadelphia, WB Saunders, 1980

Meislin, HW: Priorities in multiple trauma. Top Emerg Med, 1:1–157, 1979

Molyneux-Luick M, Knecht JW: The emergency that supersedes all other duties: Hypovolemic shock. Nursing '77, 7:32–35, 1977

Murray J, Smallwood J: CVP monitoring: Sidestepping potential perils. Nursing '77, 7:41–47, 1977

Ransom K, McSwain NE: Respiratory function following application of MAST trousers. J Am Coll Emerg Phys, 7:297–299, 1978

Rockwood CA, Mann CM, Farrington JD, et al.: History of emergency medical services in the United States. J Trauma, 16:299–308, 1976

Rutherford E: The trauma team concept in a rural hospital. Handout, Central Washington Health Services Consortium, Wenatchee, Washington, June, 1974

Shaw RK, Ariyan S, Krant SM, et al.: Modifications in the treatment of the multiple injury patient. J Trauma, 17:630–633, 1977

Shires GT, Black EA eds.: Consensus development conference. Supportive

Therapy in Burn Care. Proceedings of a conference at the National Institutes of Health, Bethesda, Maryland, 10–11 November, 1978. J Trauma, (Suppl), 19:855–939, 1979

Stürm A, Lewis FR, Trentz O, et al.: Cardiopulmonary parameters and prognosis after severe multiple trauma. J Trauma, 19:305–318, 1979

Tintinalli JE; Tibial compartment syndrome. J Am Coll Emerg Phys, 6:506–507, 1977

Tullis JL: Albumin. I. Background and use. JAMA, 237:355–360, 1977

Tullis JL: Albumin. II. Guidelines for clinical use. JAMA, 237:460–463, 1977

Wilson RF, Wilson JA: Pathophysiology, diagnosis, and treatment of shock. J Emerg Nurs, 3:11–16, 1977

Index

Page numbers followed by f represent figures; page numbers followed by t represent tables

117